CHRISTINE MCMAHON SUTTON

STOP AND SMELL THE GARBAGE

A Caregiver's Story of Survival

Stop and Smell the Garbage

A Caregiver's Story of Survival

Christine McMahon Sutton
caregiver822@gmail.com

Cover photo by Christine McMahon Sutton

ISBN - 13: 978-1477574072
ISBN - 10: 1477574077

For Gery, who had enough courage for us both

Our walking path took us past a large garbage can that sat near an apartment complex. It was a favorite stopping point for dogs and Lucy, our willful terrier, pulled me over to it. I asked, "Oh, do you want to stop and smell the garbage?"

Gery didn't appear to be paying attention, but not only was he listening, he decided I was talking to him. He walked resolutely to the garbage can, removed the lid, lowered his head and took an enthusiastic whiff.

At age fifty-six, Gery Sutton—a family physician who specialized in geriatric medicine—was diagnosed with early onset Alzheimer's. For three years, his wife was his full time caregiver. Because nothing in her background prepared her, she did what most caregivers do—she made it up as she went along. This is her forthright account of the daily challenges, the failures and the unexpected triumphs. She gives realistic advice on caring for someone with dementia. She describes signs of Alzheimer's that she saw and misinterpreted during the months before her husband's diagnosis. She shares the coping mechanisms that helped her survive the illness and death of her husband. Finally, she describes her search for meaning at the bottom of a garbage can.*

*The garbage can on the book cover is the same one referred to in the above passage.

Stop and Smell the Garbage

Contents *A Caregiver's Story of Survival*

The voice of a caregiver

When my husband was diagnosed with early onset Alzheimer's, I acquired a number of advice books. Although the authors were well-intentioned and I craved advice, I had difficulty reading them. My attention span was so ravaged by stress and depression that I wasn't able to concentrate.

Sometimes I managed to read a page or two, but was left feeling frustrated and alienated. It seemed as if no one was talking about how it really feels to be a caregiver.

When I complained to my friends, they said, "You're a writer. Write your own book."

I liked this idea and began making occasional notes. I didn't know what form my book would take, I knew only that I wanted to write the advice book I wish someone had given to me. A book in a caregiver-friendly format. A book that honestly addresses caregivers' feelings. A book that places caregivers and those they care for on an equal footing. A book that doesn't blink in the face of reality.

I wanted to write a book that honestly addresses the feelings of caregivers. A book that places caregivers on an equal footing.

Alzheimer's is a single diagnosis that encompasses a wide variety of symptoms and behaviors, many of which are not well-understood. The manifestations of this disease in your loved one may be totally different from those I observed in my husband. When you've seen one Alzheimer's patient, you've seen one Alzheimer's patient.

For example, my husband never became violent or belligerent, though I was warned this was likely. However, he displayed anxiety advancing dementia. In those terrible dark hours when sleep was impossible, I had thoughts that frightened me.

The future seemed so ominous that I wished something would happen to us—a fatal car crash, for example—so we would be spared the ordeal ahead. Sometimes I wished God would take Gery and spare him the terrible disintegration of his brain.

I had never experienced emotions like these. Getting out of bed to face the day was almost physically painful. I moved in slow motion. I felt heavy, as if I'd collapsed in on myself. Depression is relentlessly self-absorbed. Though Gery was the one with a terminal illness, I was consumed by my own pain.

Desperate to escape the terrible feelings, I asked our family physician for antidepressants. One pill intensified the teeth-grinding that had already left me with two cracked molars. Two weeks of pills made me feel oddly fuzzy but no less depressed. Then I began to gain weight, which exacerbated the arthritis in my knees and hips.

Disgusted, I quit the pills. Being depressed was bad enough; depressed and overweight was unthinkable. If they can't find an effective Alzheimer's treatment, can't they at least invent an antidepressant that doesn't pile on the pounds?

Depression is relentlessly self-absorbed. Though Gery was the one with the terminal illness, I was consumed by my own pain.

A neurologist at the Mayo Clinic said something that marked the start of my ascent from the depths. I requested a private meeting with him so I could ask questions I didn't want Gery to hear. The doctor asked how I was coping, then surprised me by inquiring if I had thoughts of what he called *passive suicide*. He described this as wishing something catastrophic would happen to one or both of us. My throat was so constricted I could only nod in the affirmative. He patted my shoulder. "Perfectly normal," he said. "It will pass."

Maybe I was tired of feeling wretched, or maybe he caught me at the right time for another reason. I left the room feeling a bit better, a bit lighter. A physician—and an acknowledged Alzheimer's expert—said my feelings were normal. Knowing others shared these shameful thoughts neutralized some of their power.

Later I remembered something Gery said the day we got the awful news. The neurologist had asked him if he was a suicide risk. It was an understandable question under the circumstances, but Gery was shocked. "I don't know why he asked me that," he said later that evening. "How could he think I'd do that to people?"

I kept silent at the time, but the more I thought about his reaction, the more I was ashamed of myself. Gery's profession robbed him of the gift of ignorance. As a geriatric specialist, he knew exactly what he was facing. Even in the wake of the worst possible medical news, he was able to choose life without a second's hesitation. His bravery deserved more from me, and I began to make a conscious effort to at least appear cheerful.

Nearly a year passed before I shook the hopelessness. The sadness is more intractable, but I've learned sadness and hope can coexist. Unlike depression, sadness leaves room for other feelings.

I hope I will never repeat the experience, but there is great potential value in hitting bottom. It's an opportunity to learn something about yourself and your ability to cope with tragedy. When I lost all hope, I was granted an awesome and terrible clarity that I knew could focus my vision or blind me forever. British prime minister Winston Churchill, who was greatly admired by my husband, wrote, "The glory of light cannot exist without shadows."

If you're in the dark, if you're at the bottom, please believe that hope will dawn again. It will light your path forward.▼

Remember. . . Despair is not the last emotion you will feel.

*When you hear
hoofbeats, think
horse, not zebra.*

THEODORE WOODWARD, MD
University of Maryland
School of Medicine

CHAPTER 2

Who knew it was a zebra?

When doctors study the process of diagnosing illness, they are taught to first eliminate the *horse*, or the most common cause of the symptoms. In the world of medicine, *zebra* is slang for an illness or condition that is one of the rarest causes of the symptoms.

After Gery was diagnosed, people often asked me if I'd noticed signs that something was wrong. Alzheimer's is a universally feared disease that mysteriously robs its victims of their personhood and ability to function. People want reassurance that their forgetfulness is normal, not a precursor of the unthinkable.

The first few times I was asked, I could offer no insights beyond mundane stories of lost keys and ATM cards. The response was almost always the same: a nervous laugh, followed by, "I do that!"

Gery's reputation for forgetfulness worked against him when the disease began to show.

Obviously, people who don't have dementia forget things. This is why I didn't once consider that Gery might have Alzheimer's or another neurological disease. Gery was relatively young and had none of the accepted risk factors. With the possible exception of his paternal grandmother, who died at age ninety-four, there was no known Alzheimer's in his family. There was just no reason to fear the zebra. In the aftermath of Gery's illness, I imagine his sisters are afraid it's Alzheimer's every time they forget something.

With the passage of time, I've been able to reflect more objectively on the months leading up to Gery's diagnosis. A clearer picture has emerged. In retrospect I see that he showed very real signs of the

CHAPTER 3

The reality of Alzheimer's

In 2011, a *Des Moines Register* columnist interviewed me for a story on Gery and early onset Alzheimer's. Later, I got an email from a woman whose husband was newly-diagnosed with early onset Alzheimer's. She said he had been prescribed medications but that no follow-up appointments were scheduled.

"What should we do now?" she asked.

It's been over one hundred years since Alzheimer's was first discovered, but precious little has been learned. Experts don't know what causes it or triggers it. They don't know how it destroys the brain. They don't know why symptoms vary so widely from one person to the next. They don't know why Alzheimer's progresses rapidly in some people and slowly in others. They can't definitively diagnose Alzheimer's without dissecting the brain autopsy.

The human brain is the most complex structure in the known universe, and modern medicine knows less about it than about any other part of the body.

Some people question whether early detection is a good investment when there is no effective treatment.

At the 2011 International Alzheimer's Conference in Paris, world-renowned experts engaged in an impromptu and revealing debate over the best use of research funds. Scientists are working to develop tests that detect Alzheimer's much sooner, but some attendees questioned whether early detection is the proper place to invest time and money when there is no effective treatment.

Promising research is underway, but public health experts say we are largely unprepared for the epidemic of Alzheimer's that lies ahead. Actor David Hyde Pierce, spokesperson for the National Alzheimer's Association, calls Alzheimer's "a ticking time bomb in the heads of people of my generation."

The standard of care for Alzheimer's treatment is a family of drugs called *cholinesterase inhibitors*. These drugs supposedly slow the progression of the disease. Medical literature says the drugs are most effective in the early stages of the disease and have a mild and temporary effect in approximately one-third of patients.

There are physicians who believe Alzheimer's medications are effective for some people; other physicians are openly skeptical. In an entry on the blog *Alzheimer's Reading Room*, Dr. Ira Rosofsky said that the effect of one widely used Alzheimer's drug "may be only marginally better than garlic was against the Black Death in the 14th century."

He may be right, but no one likes telling patients that modern medicine has nothing to offer, and most people don't want to hear it, especially when they are still in shock over the diagnosis. Any treatment—even an ineffective one—is better than none at all.

Gery wanted to stop one of the drugs because it caused gastrointestinal symptoms that embarrassed him.

Gery was on two Alzheimer's medications from the day he was diagnosed. His neurologist discontinued the medications when he went into long term care. Early in his illness, Gery wanted to stop one of the drugs because it caused gastrointestinal symptoms that embarrassed him. I asked him to keep taking the drug, but later I wished I had let him make his own decision. If he received any benefit from the medication, it was minimal and not worth trading his comfort and dignity. I think Gery knew it.

After Gery's diagnosis, he continued to see our family physician for routine matters and check-ups. We saw a neurologist for management of symptoms related to Alzheimer's.

I think it's a good idea to schedule appointments with your neurologist at least every six months, and more often if you feel the need. Regular appointments with the specialist will help you feel less alone as the disease progresses and your job as caregiver becomes more challenging. Your family physician and neurologist will also be valuable resources if the time comes to consider long-term care.

Remember. . .The attainable miracle is keeping your loved one as comfortable and as happy as possible.

Once you accept the reality of this disease, there is only one goal that makes sense: keeping your loved one as comfortable and happy as possible during the time that is left. It's the best goal under less-than-ideal circumstances. The happiness component will be largely up to you with help from family and friends. Keeping your loved one comfortable will require the assistance of health care professionals.

There are reasonably effective medications for treating symptoms of Alzheimer's such as anxiety, hostility, depression and sleep disturbances. Increasingly, non-drug interventions such as music or relaxation therapy are also used to ease these symptoms.

Effective management of Alzheimer's symptoms can significantly improve the quality of your spouse's life and your life as a caregiver. Without interventions to control Gery's sleep disturbances and anxiety, the quality of Gery's life would have been much worse and I may not have lasted three years as his caregiver. ▼

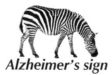
Alzheimer's sign

Gery began having problems accessing his email and his patients' electronic medical records.

Everything in life has purpose. There are no mistakes or coincidences. All events are blessings given to us to learn from.

ELIZABETH KUBLER ROSS
psychiatrist and author of *On Death and Dying*

CHAPTER 4

Stop and smell the garbage

One day toward the end of Gery's time at home, he and I were walking our dog Lucy. I held her leash since Gery could no longer handle it. We followed our usual route, which took us through a group of apartment buildings before we got to a concrete path for walkers and bikers. As always, I stared ahead at a yellow sign posted at the entrance to the path which said 'Bumps on Trail'. The sign was placed there by the city when walkers complained about the uneven concrete, but I couldn't help wondering who thought I needed a regular reminder of the bumpy course our lives had taken.

We approached a garbage can that sat near the apartment complex, a favorite stopping point for dogs. Lucy, a willful terrier, pulled me over to it. I followed her and asked, "Oh, do you want to stop and smell the garbage?"

Gery didn't appear to be paying attention, but not only was he listening, he decided I was talking to him. He walked resolutely to the garbage can, removed the lid, lowered his head and took an enthusiastic whiff.

Gery walked resolutely to the garbage can, removed the lid, lowered his head and took an enthusiastic whiff.

I drew in a shocked breath and then burst out laughing at this hilarious reminder of how literally Alzheimer's patients sometimes interpret the words they hear. It was the funniest thing Gery did during his illness and I originally intended to use it in the chapter about the humorous aspects of Alzheimer's. Then, in the coming months, this incident began to assume a new and deeper meaning.

About six months before Gery died, I was sitting with him in the nursing home when a flash of awareness miraculously worked its way through the fog. He looked directly at me and, sounding like the Gery of old, said, "It's unclear why this has happened to us."

When I recovered from my shock at encountering a Gery I thought was lost forever, I thought about what he had said. Countless times, I'd asked myself why. Gery was a good man doing good work. Why was he taken from us while evil people prospered? Why did fate dump on us? An event this colossally unfair deserved an explanation beyond random biology.

Eventually, I grew weary of the intellectual head-banging, and I realized that knowing why wouldn't make losing Gery one bit easier to bear. Over time, my grudging acceptance cleared the way for an unexpected realization. Where there is no why, there can still be meaning. Even in a pile of stinky garbage.

Look closer. Find the meaning.

Around the time Gery was diagnosed with Alzheimer's, the husband of a dear friend also got a devastating diagnosis—bone cancer. Chuck was too ill to be left alone at home, but Connie had to continue working as a teacher and needed a caregiver for Chuck while she was at work. She asked if Gery would sit with Chuck.

Gery and Chuck had much in common. Both of their fathers had been physicians. Both were in happy second marriages to their high school sweethearts. Both were facing a terminal illness with pragmatic courage.

Gery sat with Chuck a few days each week. They got along well and seemed comfortable with each other. I believe Connie felt better with Gery there because, early in his illness, he still retained much of his medical knowledge.

Eventually, Chuck became so ill that he was hospitalized much of the time and Gery's help was no longer needed.

Gery and Chuck were on separate journeys to the same destination.

Briefly, they traveled together and it was a good thing for both of them. I hope Chuck felt less alone; I know Gery felt less useless.

Look closer. Find the meaning.

Among Gery's possessions are several manila envelopes filled with letters and cards from patients, and photos of babies he delivered. The letters are a tribute to Gery's skill and empathy. They are tangible evidence of the lives he touched as a physician.

Gery continued to touch lives after he became ill. Everyone who came into contact with him was affected in a positive way. His participation in a drug trial contributed to our knowledge about Alzheimer's. He was the youngest dementia patient ever admitted to the nursing home, and the staff told me they learned from him every day he was a resident there.

Look closer. Find the meaning.

I was determined that Gery would donate his tissue and optic nerves because I saw it as a way something good could come from the nightmare of his illness. In the end, he died of a septic infection and couldn't donate. However, the staff at the state donor network—who worked very hard to help me form a plan for donation—told me they learned something new about organ and tissue donation because of my refusal to take no for an answer.

Look closer. Find the meaning.

Have you ever wondered how you would handle a terminal illness? Gery's behavior couldn't have been more admirable. He consciously chose happiness and optimism every day. He recognized false hope and refused to waste time on it. Even when he was in a pitiful state physically and mentally, he was still smiling. It was remarkable. We had the rare privilege of watching someone face a terminal illness with amazing grace and courage. More than one person voiced the hope that in a similar situation, they would be

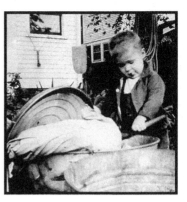

GERY, AGE 3

half as brave as Gery. I believe many people will remember his amazing courage.

Look closer. Find the meaning.

Though the doctors told us the disease had been coming on for decades, we had been married just five years when Gery was diagnosed. Our time together was sadly brief, and Gery's illness is the worst thing that has happened to someone I love, but I learned from it. I learned that the only security in life is your own inner strength. I learned that a few years with the right person are infinitely better than a lifetime with the wrong one. I learned that it is a rare and precious gift when someone loves you selflessly, with no agenda beyond your happiness. I learned that people who treat loved ones badly or take them for granted do so at their peril, because anyone can be taken away in a heartbeat.

One of Gery's nursing home caregivers told me something so wonderful I will never forget it. "I can't ever be angry at my husband over something trivial," she said. "All I do is think of you and Gery."

This book is my last love letter to my husband. Writing it soothed my aching heart and strengthened my conviction that Gery and I were brought together for a reason. If our story eases the burden of other caregivers, if it helps them in one small way, we will have found the most wonderful gift of all buried at the bottom of the garbage can.▼

Bad news isn't wine.
It doesn't improve
with age.

GENERAL COLIN POWELL
former US Secretary of State

CHAPTER 5

Communicating the right message

When someone is diagnosed with Alzheimer's, deciding who to tell, when to tell and how to tell is difficult. It's a decision with far-reaching ramifications.

Gery and I decided that our immediate family, our siblings and our closest friends should be told right away. We didn't want to take the chance they would hear it from someone else. It was emotionally draining, but we shared the news with all of them within a few days of learning Gery's diagnosis.

After that came the task of deciding who else to tell and how to do it. The correct answer to that question was much less obvious.

I have heard of people who never publicly admitted that their family member had Alzheimer's. Of course, everyone knew. We live in a small town. Patient confidentiality laws aren't always respected and people like to gossip. It's not motivated by maliciousness, it's just human nature. When there is bad news to be told, even a city can seem a lot like a small town. People can hear the truth from you, or they will hear a version of the truth from the rumor mill.

Not being honest sends a negative message: *We're ashamed and we don't trust you with the truth.*

I believe that not being honest about Alzheimer's sends a very negative message to friends and acquaintances: *We're ashamed and we don't trust you with the truth.*

An obvious reason for not wanting an Alzheimer's diagnosis to be generally known is how it might affect employment. However, by the time Alzheimer's is diagnosed, the person has often been put on

CHAPTER 6

A day without Alzheimer's

Once, late in his illness, Gery informed me earnestly that he no longer believed he had Alzheimer's. I was happy to agree that he had been misdiagnosed. "Damn those doctors anyway!" I exclaimed. "What do they know?"

I can't recall another occasion when I heard Gery make a direct reference to having Alzheimer's. His failure to discuss or even mention his terrible diagnosis was eerie. I assumed he was in deep denial or that his dementia was already so advanced he had forgotten he had Alzheimer's.

I would have been happy to discuss Gery's illness with him if he had broached the topic. I couldn't believe that he didn't want to talk about it. I came close to bringing it up several times, but something stopped me. I took my cue from Gery and never said the A word when we were together.

I assumed he was in deep denial or that his dementia was already so advanced he had forgotten he had Alzheimer's.

After Gery went to the nursing home, surprising stories began trickling back to me. People reported hearing Gery joke about his illness. When someone lost a set of keys or an ATM card, Gery laughed and said, "Hey, I'm the one with Alzheimer's!"

I learned that he had spoken frankly to his sister about his illness, telling her he was worried about whether I would be OK after he was gone. He said he was counting on "the family guys" to help me.

Then came a story that truly shocked me. On their way to lunch one day, Gery told his friend John, "I have five years if I'm lucky."

When I expressed astonishment because Gery hadn't once said anything like this to me, John replied, "He didn't want to upset you."

At that moment, I knew I had completely misinterpreted Gery's earlier reticence on the topic of Alzheimer's. Obviously, he made a decision not to mention it to me. By not talking about it, he thrust aside the hideous specter of a terminal disease to make way for normalcy. My wise and pragmatic husband understood what I didn't: talking about it would have been painful and pointless. What I thought was denial or dementia was an act of selflessness. It was Gery's wonderful gift to us.

Remember. . . The person with the terminal illness should decide whether or not you discuss it.

I don't recommend that you refuse to discuss the Alzheimer's or the cancer or the ALS if your spouse wants to. I don't recommend that you force the issue. I'm advising you to follow your loved one's lead. The person with the terminal illness should decide.

My husband taught me it is a victory of immense proportions just to spend the day together, occupied by normal pursuits and mundane concerns. You'll own the day forever because you snatched it from the elephant in the room and made it your own.

For just one day, the disease didn't win.▼

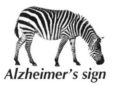

Alzheimer's sign

In twenty-six years of practice, Gery was never sued and I had never heard him express a fear of being sued. Suddenly, he was convinced a patient was about to sue him. When he told me the details of the case, I felt his concern was baseless. For several days, he brought it up repeatedly. Nothing I said reassured him.

Live every day as if
it were your last.
Someday, you'll
be right.

HH 'BREAKER' MORANT
Australian army officer
executed in 1902 for
following orders

CHAPTER 7

The long goodbye may not be so long

The only time I asked one of Gery's doctors how long he might live, I was told he could trundle along in passable condition for twelve to fifteen years. That estimate proved to be wildly optimistic, but I am grateful for it. At that moment, it was what I needed to hear.

Predicting longevity is a dicey business. Many physicians see it as a no-win because they will almost certainly be quoted when they're wrong and less often when they're right.

Understandably, the life expectancy question is the one nearly everyone asks when diagnosed with a terminal illness. When the illness is Alzheimer's, the answer seems particularly elusive.

In 2010, a physician developed a formula for predicting how long someone will live with Alzheimer's. He created it after noticing the wide disparity in longevity among his Alzheimer's patients, some living just a few years and others as long as twenty years. His formula is based on three factors: gender (men fare worse), level of impairment at the time of diagnosis and age at diagnosis. The formula's age component presupposes that the younger you are when you are diagnosed, the longer you will live.

Experts say people spend forty percent of their years with Alzheimer's in the final stage of the disease.

After Gery's diagnosis, I heard many stories about people with early onset Alzheimer's. If Gery wasn't within earshot, I asked how long the person lived and the answers were disheartening, to say the least. Three years. One year. In one notable case, six months. I began to wonder if the Alzheimer's in people under age sixty-five is

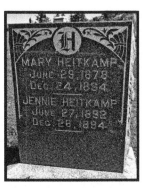

THE SAD HEADSTONE

Their parents, memorialized on the other side of the headstone, had outlived their daughters by decades.

"What do you suppose they died of?" I asked the first day we noticed it.

"Whatever childhood epidemic was going around that winter," Gery replied.

I still walk the same trail, and each time I pass that headstone I think about the unspeakable tragedy that life dealt those parents on that long ago Christmas. I feel the impotent rage of losing a loved one to a disease that will be preventable or treatable someday. I feel the despair of losing someone you love way too soon.

Mostly, I contemplate the fragility and the preciousness of life. Time can be your mortal enemy, but it can also be your faithful friend. You have the power to decide.▼

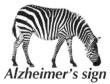

Alzheimer's sign

Gery was part of a seventy-physician primary care group, and his compensation included a salary and a quarterly bonus based on productivity. Gery carefully checked each bonus for accuracy. He often called the administrative office to question a calculation. In 2006, his bonus began to decline. When I asked him why, he had no explanation and seemed disinterested.

*If misery loves
company, then
misery has
company enough.*

HENRY DAVID THOREAU
American author
and philosopher

CHAPTER 8

Thanks for sharing

I've never been much of a joiner, but when someone told me about a new support group for people with early onset Alzheimer's and their caregivers in a town fifteen miles away, we decided to attend a meeting.

The group leaders were very warm and welcoming. After introductions, we were divided into two groups—people with Alzheimer's and caregivers. The caregiver group moderator was a lovely woman whose husband had died of early onset Alzheimer's several years earlier. She seemed sad and a little subdued, but sane and functioning. It encouraged me to see someone who made it through to the other side of caregiving.

However, after an hour of sharing our feelings, I knew this wasn't for me. We live in a relatively rural area, and there weren't enough younger participants. In my experience, some issues faced by people with early onset Alzheimer's are vastly different from those faced by people over age sixty-five.

I didn't want to share my feelings. I wanted practical advice from someone who had been in my situation and survived.

Hearing other people's stories didn't make me feel better or less alone, it made me feel even more depressed and stressed. I didn't want to share my feelings or hear about anyone else's feelings. I thought it was safe to assume we all felt like hell. I wanted practical advice from someone who had been in my situation and survived.

By the time we got in the car to drive home, I was in a terrible mood. I felt very sorry for a woman whose husband got red-faced and angry and made her leave in the middle of the meeting. I was disgusted with a woman who forced her husband to admit, every day, that he had Alzheimer's. I should have had more empathy for another caregiver, but she made me wonder what stupid mistakes I was making without realizing it.

It's admirable that the organizers donated their time to help us, and I know I didn't give the group a fair chance. I would have gone back if Gery had wanted to, but he said his feelings were neutral.

On our way home, I thought about things the other caregivers had said. Some of our challenges were similar, and others were different, but we all had the same shell-shocked look.

I was curious about the issues that were discussed in Gery's group, and asked him what they had talked about. Obviously annoyed, he replied, "Chris, I don't even remember what I said. How can I remember what the other people said?"

So, at the end of a not-so-great evening, Gery made me laugh. That was worth the drive.▼

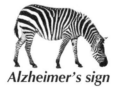

Alzheimer's sign

Gery went with me one Saturday to get groceries. Snow was predicted, and the parking lot was packed. We pushed our full cart outside and Gery told me to wait while he got the car. It was nearly twenty minutes before he appeared in our car. When I asked what had taken so long, he didn't answer and seemed very upset.

application said she wasn't sure he would qualify since he had so much education. However, our claim was approved and we began receiving a monthly check. Gery's youngest son received benefits until he turned eighteen. Gery and I were grateful recipients.

I got a job as a retail merchandiser doing product resets. The job was physically taxing, but the pay was better than minimum wage and the hours were flexible. That allowed me to drive Gery to the Mayo Clinic every six weeks to participate in the trial of a new drug.

Within six months, the dust cleared and we were living on one-tenth of our former income. Gery didn't qualify for Medicare until he had been disabled for two years; the monthly bill just for our health insurance and the Alzheimer's medications was nearly equal to the average house payment.

Within six months of Gery's diagnosis, the dust cleared and we were living on one-tenth of our former income.

We bought a house which was two blocks from the high school football field where we had spent many happy hours. An older brick home, small and charming, it had a large yard and mature trees. It was in our limited price range. Once we knew there would be enough money for the basics, we didn't mind our reduced circumstances. We had never indulged in expensive cars or other luxuries. Being at home had always been our favorite pastime.

Less than a year after Gery's diagnosis, it was obvious that he was deteriorating more rapidly than I had hoped. It was only a matter of time before he couldn't be left alone and, without my salary, we would be unable to pay our bills.

I was contacted by a woman I had worked with at the state medical society. She wanted to start a freelance business providing services for physician specialty groups. It was a great opportunity, and by the time I had to quit my job we had two clients. I could work at home and Gery would be safe.

What early onset Alzheimer's cost us

Thirteen years of lost income*	$2,925,000
Nursing home (15 months)	$70,426
Gery's COBRA insurance 2008-09	$8,723
Chris health insurance 2008-11	$8,624
Alzheimer's medications (co-pays)	$4,078
Alzheimer's doctor visits (co-pays)	$2,096
Ten trips to Mayo Clinic	$1,500
TOTAL DIRECT COSTS	$3,020,447

*Assumes retirement at age 68, though it's likely Gery would have worked longer

The biggest remaining hurdle was the cost of long term care. We had discussed purchasing long term care insurance but decided to wait until we were older. Now, it was too late. I did some research and learned that Title 19 would pay for long term care after we exhausted Gery's 401(k).

When Gery went to the nursing home, I paid the monthly bill from his retirement fund. I had enough money for two more months when he died. I was spared the ordeal of applying for Title 19 assistance.

Though Gery was in a nursing home, he was also a hospice patient. Medicare paid for visits from hospice staff and for comfort medications such as anti-anxiety medications and muscle relaxants.

During the last two years of his illness, his advanced dementia made it impossible for him to participate in financial decisions. Even early in his illness, his anxiety was palpable when he was expected to deal with a financial or legal issue. I began using his power of attorney for business when he could no longer talk with people on the phone, sign his name or understand the issue at hand.

I called every company we dealt with for goods and services and said I would be acting on Gery's behalf. All the companies required that I send a copy of my power of attorney for their files. Several companies also asked for a letter from Gery's doctor. An illness such as Alzheimer's generates a sea of paperwork.

My experience married to someone with Alzheimer's taught me that the legal and financial issues are complex and require guidance from the very best professionals. I have three final pieces of advice:

• SEE AN ATTORNEY

You and your spouse each need up-to-date wills, living wills and powers of attorney for health care decisions. You each need to designate a power of attorney for business as well. Do this as soon as possible. Make plenty of copies of all documents. Some people in our situation obtain a legal guardianship. Your attorney must be the one to advise you on these issues, based on your particular circumstances and the laws in your state.

• SEE A FINANCIAL ADVISOR

A terminal illness changes everything in your financial world. An illness that involves dementia raises particularly knotty issues. See a financial advisor as soon as you can and plan for the worst case scenario. Make sure the financial advisor understands your altered circumstances, goals and timeframes. I spoke privately with the planner before our appointment because I couldn't speak frankly about Gery's prognosis and its implications when he was present.

• CHECK THAT WALLET OR PURSE

Shortly after Gery was diagnosed with Alzheimer's, he handed me his credit card and said, "I don't think I should have this." In the coming weeks, he lost his wallet and misplaced his ATM card numerous times. I became concerned about the security of our accounts. I asked him if he wanted to start carrying more cash, and how much he wanted. He said, "Fifty dollars." I put the money in his wallet and, without saying anything to him, took his ATM card. He never asked about the card. Until his dementia became severe, he always had fifty dollars in his wallet.▼

*The fact that the mind
rules the body is the most
fundamental fact we
know about the
process of life.*

FRANZ ALEXANDER, MD
founder of
psychosomatic medicine

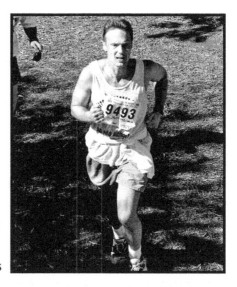

**GERY IN THE
MARINE CORPS
MARATHON, 1995**

never actually seen someone have a seizure, but that's the best word I can use to describe the rhythmic jerking and tremors that contorted his whole body. I witnessed many of these episodes but, other than keep him from falling out of bed, there wasn't much I could do but watch. Like other manifestations of Alzheimer's, I got used to it.

Gery resisted the idea of a bedrail, but I insisted after he fell out of bed and cut his face on the nightstand. The bedrail solved that problem, but, as often happens with Alzheimer's, it caused another one. Gery had trouble maneuvering around the bedrail when he had to go to the bathroom at night. The first time he was incontinent, the bedrail was a factor.

By the time Gery finished the clinical trial, the seizures were more frequent and intense. His neurologist ordered a CAT scan, which showed no seizure activity. The doctor told me these episodes were not seizures because people can't be roused from seizures. He said that clonazepam was the appropriate treatment.

I told him Gery was unaware of these sleep episodes and that I didn't want to worry him by discussing it. I asked if I could give him the medication without discussing it with him. The neurologist wasn't comfortable with this plan. I understand the importance of patient autonomy, but I knew what would happen. Gery looked very frightened when the doctor spoke with him about the seizures. On the way home, his hands shook. "If that's happening at night, I'm afraid pretty soon I won't be able to do things during the day," he said. There was fear in his voice and, despite my reassurances, he brought it up several times over the next few days.

The clonazepam resolved the problem, but then his arms and legs began trembling when he was awake. One morning a few months before he went to the nursing home, his left arm began twitching violently as he walked through the living room. He looked terrified.

Some of Gery's caregivers believed anxiety was the cause of the muscle tremors. I think this was true early in his illness, but I suspect the firestorm in his brain was the culprit in the advanced stages of the disease. During the last month of his life, Gery's neck muscles knotted so violently that his face was a mask of pain. Our physician prescribed a morphine derivative that relieved his discomfort.

Even early in his illness, Gery stumbled and tripped fairly often. One day, he was sweeping the carpet and tripped over the vacuum cleaner cord. He fell very hard and broke a small table in the hallway. It upset him a great deal, and it was one of many times I felt so sorry for him I thought my heart would break.

Before I realized that a disintegrating brain sends faulty signals to the arms and legs, I let Gery do things that put him at risk for accidents. I shouldn't have let him climb a ladder to get sticks off the roof or carry boxes down the basement stairs.

As a caregiver, I frequently felt that the disease was winning the race. Just when I solved one Alzheimer's riddle, another appeared. Literally and figuratively, Gery's physical symptoms were another illustration of my original title for this book — "One Step Behind."▼

Remember. . . Alzheimer's can affect coordination and balance.

*For some, losing driving
privileges causes a
stronger grief reaction
than the diagnosis of
Alzheimer's.*

Leilani Doty, PhD
University of Florida
Cognitive and Memory Disorder Clinics

CHAPTER 11

Keeper of the keys

An Alzheimer's diagnosis raises many tough issues. Though driving is one of the toughest, I felt we had to deal with it as soon as Gery was diagnosed. I had heard too many stories about people with Alzheimer's who were found three states away with no memory of driving anywhere.

There are doctors who advise patients to stop driving the same day they deliver the diagnosis of Alzheimer's; other doctors don't address the issue unless asked to. In any case, you're the one who must help your loved one adjust to this loss of independence.

Even my normally compliant husband became surprisingly mulish on this topic. I felt awful bringing it up because I already felt so sorry for him. I gently suggested that he think about not driving anymore, but he argued that there were drivers more impaired than he was, especially in a town with many elderly people.

He argued that there were drivers more impaired than he was, especially in a town with many elderly people.

He was right, but I knew I couldn't compromise on the issue of highway driving. Gery's early symptoms showed in his driving abilities, and he wasn't able to handle a car at high speeds. I tried hard to make it sound temporary.

"Why don't you try driving just in town for the time being," I said. He reluctantly agreed. He continued driving in town for nearly a year. Then he got a ticket for failure to yield. He was so distraught he was almost in tears. I said the ticket was no big deal. I suggested we pay it and move on. The woman at the courthouse said no one

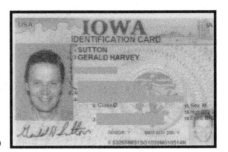

GERY'S PHOTO ID

had ever come that quickly to pay a hundred dollar ticket.

I asked him to drive me to the store so I could observe him behind the wheel. What I saw wasn't encouraging. I called his neurologist, and, at our next appointment, he told Gery he couldn't continue driving unless he passed the driving test.

We got the driving manual and for several days, Gery studied for the written portion of the exam. He took the practice test over and over, never scoring above fifty percent. He became increasingly frustrated. Finally, I asked him as gently as I could if he thought this was a good use of his time. His shoulders sagged. "No," he said.

The next day, we went to the courthouse again. Gery surrendered his driver's license and got an identification card. He joked with the women behind the counter and winked at me right before they snapped his photo. I've never loved him more than I loved him in that moment. That identification card will always be a tangible reminder of my husband's amazing courage.

A friend gave him a red bicycle we named the Pee-Wee Herman bike. He seemed content to pedal around town and he became quite fond of that bicycle. Eventually, he stopped riding on his own. I'm not sure why.▼

Remember. . . Consult your physician
about the issue of Alzheimer's and driving.

If you don't like something, change it. If you can't change it, change the way you think about it.

MARY ENGELBREIT
children's book
illustrator

CHAPTER 12

Hats, purses and potato salad

It's hard to imagine living in a universe with no rules and no order, but that's what it means to have Alzheimer's. As the disease progresses, a lifetime of accumulated knowledge about everyday living is inexorably destroyed. Learned associations fade, leaving an existential world full of objects and people whose purpose and meaning are no longer instinctively clear.

I vividly remember the first time Gery did something bizarre. For six months after his diagnosis, the signs of Alzheimer's had pretty much stayed within the boundaries of extreme forgetfulness, lack of initiative, clinginess and an inability to concentrate. Then one day, he emerged from the bedroom smiling and wearing three baseball caps neatly stacked one on top of the other. Horrified, I took refuge in the bathroom and sobbed quietly into a towel.

If he wanted to put on five pairs of socks or walk the dog to the end of the block ten times in one morning, who was he hurting?

There were days when I would have traded Gery's Alzheimer's for just about any other illness if it would have spared us the relentless deterioration of his brain. I was powerless to stop it. Being a full time eye witness to his downhill slide felt like torture.

Of course, the whacky behavior became more frequent and then became the rule rather than the exception. As time went on, I also experienced a mental transformation. Mercifully, my overheated reaction gave way to pragmatism. I would never have thought it possible, but I actually got used to it. With a couple of exceptions, nothing he did shocked or even surprised me. If he wanted to put on five pairs of socks and walk the dog to the end of the block ten times in one morning, who was he hurting? I was the only one upset. The biggest problem was prying off the multiple layers of socks.

When Gery carefully assembled a potato salad sandwich at a dinner with friends, I didn't experience that sick feeling in the pit of my stomach. Someone said later that the sandwich looked good. When Gery was out of earshot, we joked about compiling a book of creative food pairings from Alzheimer's patients.

Remember. . . You'll be amazed by what you can get used to.

On one occasion, Gery did something that upset him. We were leaving a funeral luncheon, and a woman ran after us calling "Sir! Sir!" in an agitated voice. Gery had picked up her purse, which was the same color as mine. The woman grabbed it out of his hand with an annoyed sniff and stalked off.

As we drove home, Gery's hands shook and he looked on the verge of tears. "Why did I do that?" he asked. "That woman must think I'm crazy!"

I hated seeing him so upset. I quickly reassured him that anyone could make the same mistake. I called the woman "stupid and rude" for thinking he was stealing her handbag. My attitude immediately changed his and later, he joked about the incident.

"Maybe purse-snatching can be my new career," he said with a rueful grin.

"You'd better practice because you're not very good at it," I advised and Gery laughed.▼

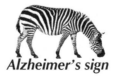

Alzheimer's sign

I noticed Gery was very quiet in social situations, rarely speaking. I asked him if he needed to have his hearing checked but he said no.

*Insanity is doing
the same thing
over and over
and expecting
a different result.*

ALBERT EINSTEIN
father of modern physics

CHAPTER 13

Don't be a repeat machine

Early in Gery's illness, he asked me the same questions over and over and over. What day is it? What date is it? What time are we going to Bob and Susan's house? What did you want from the basement? Sometimes he pretended that he hadn't heard my answer the first or second time, but he abandoned that tactic when I began urging him to have his hearing checked.

At first, before I understood the problem, I assumed it was my fault for not making my answers clear enough for Gery to understand. The almost irresistible temptation was to keep repeating the same answer. I said it louder, more succinctly. I rearranged the words, saying them in every possible order. I used different words. I told myself that this time he'll understand and not ask again. Wrong! He asked the same question as many times as I would answer it.

I was sucked into the Repetition Vortex way too often, causing myself untold stress and frustration.

I was sucked into the Repetition Vortex way too often, causing myself untold stress and frustration. Why had I suddenly become a poor communicator? Why couldn't I make him understand? Finally, I had to face reality: the part of my husband's brain that processed language was already damaged. There was no magic combination of words that would make him remember which night we were having dinner with friends, or restore his ability to perform a sequential task such as running the dishwasher.

I tried a new strategy. Because Gery repeatedly asked about our social engagements, I posted a list on the refrigerator titled "This

Week." It listed each day, the activities scheduled for that day and the time of each activity. I wrote with a felt tip marker, in large letters and numbers.

Whenever Gery asked about our social engagements, I referred him to the refrigerator. Eventually, he went to the refrigerator schedule without questioning me first, proving that Alzheimer's patients can learn new lessons with enough repetition.

For other questions, I adopted a new policy. For the sake of my own sanity, I answered the same question no more than twice. That didn't mean he stopped asking, but when he asked a third time, I said, "You're smart. You'll figure it out." As long as you're smiling and you sound happy, any noncommittal answer should do the trick.

Remember. . . Answer a question twice, and no more.

Sometimes, when he kept repeating the same question, I smiled at him, kissed his cheek and said nothing. Occasionally that worked, or maybe it just confused him enough that he stopped asking.

There were times when none of these tactics were successful, and Gery kept repeating his question, becoming angrier and more frustrated with each repetition. One day, because I didn't know what else to do, I told him the absolute truth.

"You've asked me that question several times and I've answered it several times. If you ask me that question again, I'm going to get upset. I don't want to get upset because I think we're having a really good day and I don't want to ruin it!"

That tactic worked like a charm, and I used it often during the time Gery was still asking questions.▼

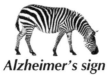

Alzheimer's sign

For the first time, one of Gery's sons beat him at chess.

Life does not cease
to be funny when
people die anymore than
it ceases to be serious
when people laugh.

GEORGE BERNARD SHAW
Irish playwright

CHAPTER 14

Crop signs from the planet amyloid*

Gery was the first to see the humor potential in Alzheimer's and, early in his illness, the jokes were on me.

A few months after his diagnosis, I was still struggling to accept the terrible implications for our future. I was depressed and mostly unable to laugh or even smile. I wasn't ready to see any humor in this awful situation. One day, I sent Gery to the grocery store for canned corn. He came home, put a grocery bag on the counter and announced cheerfully, "Here's your tomato sauce!"

I stared at him in shock. A huge grin appeared on his face and I knew he had tricked me. "You are not funny!" I told him. One morning a few weeks later, Gery announced he was going to take a shower. He shut the bathroom door and I heard the water running. Gery always took very long showers, and it was some time before I heard the water turn off. The bathroom door opened and he called, "Honey, would you come here?"

I wasn't ready to see any humor in this awful situation. I was depressed and mostly unable to laugh or even smile.

He was standing in the doorway with a towel around his waist. Drops of water glistened on his chest and his hair was soaking wet. "I'm going to take my shower now!" he said. I was horrified, and it showed. This was exactly the kind of Alzheimer's symptom I'd been dreading. Then I saw his self-satisfied smile. He'd punked me again.

"Gery Sutton, you're not funny!" I yelled and stomped off. But I

*Amyloid is a protein that collects in the brain, causing Alzheimer's.

was wrong. He was very funny. I was just too upset to appreciate it. Gery never met a pun he didn't like, and his ability to make a groan-inducing pun stayed with him for a surprisingly long time. He was watching the news when Bernie Madoff was arrested, and said, "Honey, look at this! Bernie made off with everyone's money!"

The first time I remember seeing humor in Alzheimer's was much later. Gery was doing all sorts of bizarre things, though his actions were no longer intentional. One morning after a snowstorm, he went out to shovel the sidewalk. I followed him, planning to run errands. We were looking at the drifts when, without warning, he jumped off the side of the porch, landing on the snow-covered bushes.

His action and the surprised look on his face made me grin. "What are you doing?" I asked. This was a stupid question, but for some reason I couldn't stop asking it. I helped him to his feet, and brushed the snow off him as I once did for my kids.

As I got into my car, I saw him grab a bag of ice melt and begin wildly throwing it around the yard. I rolled down the car window and called, "Looks like you're going to need a lot more of that stuff!" He smiled and waved and I drove away, laughing for the first time in months.

Gery did funny things nearly every day, but my typical reaction was shock, sadness or numb acceptance.

The ability to laugh proved to be a rare and very welcome gift. In truth, Gery did funny things nearly every day, but my typical reaction was shock, sadness or numb acceptance. I remember clearly each time I laughed because it didn't happen often.

We were visiting my son and his family in Las Vegas and, while we were there, I heard my son complain repeatedly about misplacing his toothbrush. I also misplaced my toothbrush and had to buy another. I was in the bathroom helping Gery get ready to fly back home when he opened his toiletry bag and pulled out a handful of toothbrushes. Looking completely bewildered, he fanned them out like a deck of cards. "Who do all these toothbrushes belong to?" he asked. I burst out laughing. "They're yours now!"

One day when Gery was in the nursing home, I showed him the latest photo of our grandson Hayden. Gery glanced at the picture, sniffed and said, "Little bastard." Gery so rarely used this kind of language that I burst into shocked laughter. Gery laughed with me, slapping his knee in delight.

A mowing mishap occurred about a year before Gery went to the nursing home. I had a summer cold and, after lunch, fell asleep on the couch for an hour. When I woke up, I looked out the window. While I slept, someone had mowed long, criss cross swatches in our lawn. They looked like crop signs left by drunken aliens.

I located Gery in the bedroom, methodically pulling on multiple pairs of socks. "Gery, did you mow while I was sleeping?" I asked.

He looked sheepish. "I guess you think that wasn't the best idea for me and Lucy," he responded. I gasped. "Lucy was with you? On her leash?" He nodded and I was so upset I left the room. This was not funny. It wasn't safe for Gery to run a mower. I kept Lucy on a short leash, and he easily could have run over her paw.

Gery pulled on the leash, dragging Lucy and the bunched-up rug toward the front door. The poor dog looked terrified.

Later, Gery emerged from the bedroom and announced he was taking Lucy for a walk. He hooked her leash to her collar, but she dug her claws into the rug and refused to budge. Gery pulled on the leash, dragging Lucy and the bunched-up rug toward the front door. The poor dog looked terrified and I couldn't help it, I laughed. I've never seen a dog react so negatively to the prospect of a walk. I'm sure Lucy thought there was more mowing in store.

Unsuspecting strangers sometimes got in on the fun. When Gery couldn't work anymore, he sorely missed the daily contact with people. Always one to bloom where he was planted, he developed an alternative. He watched out the front window for someone to walk by our house. When he spied someone coming, he bolted out the front door and down the sidewalk calling, "Well, hi! How are you?" Sometimes it was someone he knew; sometimes it wasn't. But every time, Gery's demeanor was that of someone joyfully greeting an old friend. The first few times he did it, I held my breath for fear he would be rudely rebuffed, but every one of the passers-by smiled and greeted him in return.

However, I could see the bewilderment on their faces as they desperately searched their memories for the identity of this amiable man who greeted them so warmly. It was hilarious, like watching an episode of *Candid Camera* in your own front yard.

When he spied someone coming, he bolted out the front door and down the sidewalk calling 'Well hi! How are you?'

My final anecdote involves the most appalling thing Gery did during his three years at home. I must accept partial responsibility for the bizarre chain of events, since I was the first one to throw toilet paper into the bathroom garbage can.

One day, because we were out of tissues, I used toilet paper to take the polish off my fingernails. I discarded the toilet paper— soaked with polish and red blotches—in the garbage can in the bathroom. Later, Gery emerged from the bathroom looking agitated. He was carrying the toilet paper.

"Honey, are you bleeding?" he asked. I hastened to reassure him that it was nail polish on the toilet paper. A week later, I redid my nails using kleenex, discarded the used tissue in the bathroom garbage can and the exact same events occurred. Gery was so upset by my supposed blood loss that I began discarding the tissue in the kitchen waste can when I did my nails. I could have given up on nail polish, but it was already too late. I had seen how Alzheimer's works. The most notable feature of this disease is loss of short term memory, but when an idea miraculously embeds itself in the brain, it can't be easily dislodged. As the new idea takes up semi-permanent residence, the Alzheimer's warps it into bizarre new forms.

A few days later, I was brushing my teeth and noticed a terrible smell coming from the bathroom waste can. I opened the lid and found the culprits—wads of brown-stained toilet paper. I got a pair of tweezers from my makeup case and gingerly transferred the used paper to the toilet. As calmly as I could, I asked Gery to put his used toilet paper in the toilet and not the garbage can. He promised cheerfully to comply.

In the coming weeks, I found soiled toilet paper in the garbage can a number of times. I stopped asking him not to do it anymore.

Then I thought of a clever way to outwit him. I emptied the waste can, washed it and hid it in the basement. I was very proud of my ingenuity. The next morning, I went into the bathroom and sat down on the toilet. Instantly, my nostrils filled with an unmistakable smell.

I turned slowly to the right. On the windowsill was a long, neat row of soiled toilet paper wads—fluffy, delicate poop blossoms, lined up and waiting to be picked. I began to chuckle as I realized this was the reason he'd been in the bathroom so long that morning.

I thank God for that laughter because this could have been a low point in my years of caregiving. If I hadn't laughed at that precise moment, I might have lost it.

Don't let anyone tell you that it's wrong to see the humor in Alzheimer's. If you fully absorb the paralyzing sadness inherent in every bizarre event, you will never survive.▼

Remember. . . Seeing the humor is a great survival tool.

I have two doctors.
My left leg,
and my right.

GM TREVELYAN
British historian

CHAPTER 15

Every walk is a power walk

Walking has always been my favorite form of exercise, and the only exercise I've been able to stick to over the long haul. However, until I became a caregiver, I had no idea of the magical power in the simple act of putting one foot in front of another.

In the years before we were married, Gery was a long distance runner. He quit after running the Boston Marathon in 2000. He told me he had fulfilled the goals he'd set for himself when he started. He told a friend he wanted to spend more time with me.

Thankfully, Gery wasn't one of those joggers who believe you're not really exercising unless you're sweating profusely. In the years before Gery went into long term care, we became dedicated walkers. Four times each week, we walked two or three miles through the city park or on the walking trail near our house.

No matter how upset, stressed or depressed I was when we left home, I always felt refreshed and renewed when we returned. In addition, walking vastly improved the quality of my sleep. I discovered this because I slept poorly when the winter weather kept us inside. I bought an indoor walking DVD but it wasn't the same.

There were benefits for Gery, too. Walking eased the anxiety that was one of his most troublesome Alzheimer's symptoms.

There were benefits for Gery, too. In the early stages of his illness, walking eased the daily anxiety that was one of his most troublesome Alzheimer's symptoms.

According to scientists, walking releases endorphins, the brain's good mood chemicals. Walking also raises body temperature, which some researchers believe has a calming effect on the human psyche, and walking reduces immune system chemicals that contribute to depression. For me, walking was at least as effective as medication in controlling depression and I liked how walking made me feel. I didn't like how I felt when I was taking an antidepressant.

According to Dog Whisperer Cesar Millan, migrating with a pack is a primal need, even for domesticated canines. Say the word 'walk' to your dog and watch the excited reaction. I believe migrating is a primal need for humans, too, but the conveniences of modern life have obscured our ancient instincts.

For stressed and depressed caregivers, there is no substitute for escaping from your four walls and communing with nature, even for just forty-five minutes. The numerous physical benefits aside, there's nothing like a brisk walk to restore a sense of normalcy and adjust your perspective.▼

Remember. . . Experts say a daily walk
is an excellent stress reliever.

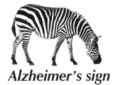

Alzheimer's sign

For years, Gery earned extra money working a monthly twelve-hour emergency room shift at a local hospital. I thought he worked way too much and urged him to quit, but he always said he couldn't afford to quit. One Sunday, he came home from the hospital and said he'd just done his last ER shift. I was so happy to have more time with my husband that I didn't ask for an explanation.

For all sad words
of tongue and pen,
the saddest are these,
It might have been.

JOHN GREENLEAF WHITTIER
Nineteenth century
American poet

CHAPTER 16

Letting go of the future

One of the most enticing aspects of marriage is the notion of growing old with someone you love. Couples in their forties and fifties begin planning for retirement, happily anticipating a time when their work and child-rearing responsibilities are behind them and they can concentrate on enjoying their lives and each other.

A terminal diagnosis is a death blow to this dream, and you'll feel the loss acutely for the foreseeable future. I may never completely lose my anger at the random unfairness of it. I suspect that I may always feel a twinge of regret and resentment when I see an elderly couple, still happily together in their eighties.

The dream of what might have been is weighty baggage on the road to the future. Though the feeling is normal, regret over my lost life with Gery has been a difficult emotion to leave behind.

I don't have a magic remedy, but I know it takes time to make an adjustment this big. Time to grieve the cozy dinners you won't have, the laughter you won't share, the vacations you won't take, the

Then and Now   Photos by Traci Clark

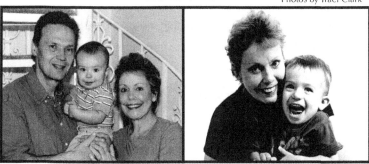

April 2010
GERY, ME AND GRANDSON HAYDEN

September 2011
ME AND GRANDSON HAYDEN

CHAPTER 17

Me and my shadow

Of all the unsettling Alzheimer's behaviors Gery exhibited during our three years at home together, there was only one that caused me intense and unrelenting annoyance. Every day, all day long, he followed me.

For the first five years of our marriage, when Gery was practicing medicine, he left home at seven a.m. and rarely returned before seven p.m. I was accustomed to being alone. However, almost from the day he was diagnosed, Gery was extremely reluctant to let me out of his sight. He was less than enthusiastic about any activity that didn't involve both of us.

Practically overnight, I went from virtual solitude to early retirement with someone who had no interests, no hobbies, no initiative and absolutely nothing to do except follow me. To say this was a difficult adjustment would be a colossal understatement.

If I went to the basement to do laundry or get my craft supplies, it was only a matter of minutes before he showed up.

If I went to the basement to do laundry or get my craft supplies, it was only a matter of minutes before he showed up. If I went into our home office to work on my computer, he followed me despite the fact that our house is very small and my office was not more than ten feet from the living room and his perch on the couch.

I tried reasoning with him as one does a child. "Gery, I'm going into my office to work for a little while. You can sit here and watch your movie. When I'm finished, we'll take a walk." This only made him feel compelled to invent an excuse for having followed me.

Some were classics, such as "Lucy looks funny." Or, "The mailman hasn't come yet."

Sometimes when he followed me, the dog followed him and the three of us formed a sad little parade. Except that it didn't make me feel sad, it made me feel so irritated and stressed I thought I might have a heart attack. One day, I burst into tears and begged him to stop following me. He looked contrite but confused.

He exhibited other behaviors that were variations on the same aggravating theme. For the first year after his diagnosis, when Gery still drove, I sent him on simple errands so I could have a blessed half hour to myself. Even this plan was flawed because he was almost incapable of actually going away. He left the house initially without a problem, but came back so many times on the flimsiest of pretexts that I could do nothing but stare at him, dumbfounded. Usually he got all the way to the car—and sometimes, inside the car —before he retraced his steps because he supposedly forgot something or needed to ask me something.

Once when I sent him to the post office for stamps, he left and returned six times before finally driving away.

Though I was mostly humor-impaired during the first year of Gery's illness, this struck me as hilariously funny. A few seconds after he left, I would hear him step back onto the porch. I amused myself by speculating on the identity of the visitor. "Who could that be?" I'd ask myself out loud. My challenge was coming up with progressively more outrageous answers. Publisher's Clearinghouse? The Avon Lady? The Fuller Brush man? Freddie Krueger?

Once when I sent him to the post office for stamps, he left and returned a record six times before finally driving away. The oddest thing was that he never exhibited the least sign of embarrassment, no matter how many return trips he made.

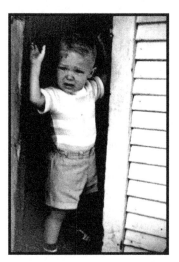

GERY, AGE 3

There was worse to come. As we sat on opposite ends of the couch, in my peripheral vision I watched his head swivel ever-so-slowly in my direction. His eyes latched onto my face and he stared, unsmiling, for so long and with such intensity that it felt, well, *creepy*. Like being stalked at very close range by a serial killer. I knew if I got up, he'd follow me, so I began shielding my face with a magazine or a notebook until he stopped staring.

The dog joined the Staring Olympics. She planted herself directly in front of me, her upward gaze boring into my forehead in a laser-like manner that is possible only if you have white fur and black eyes. Have you heard about Abbie Hoffman and his group of hippies who tried to levitate the Pentagon in the late 1960s? These two could have done it all by themselves, without the Tibetan chants.

One more variation on the follow-me theme materialized later in Gery's illness. When we went for a walk, to the grocery store or the mall, Gery walked three feet behind me. No matter how many times I asked him to walk beside me, in a few minutes he was behind me again. I tried holding his hand, but my arm wouldn't stretch that far.

I asked one of Gery's neurologists about these behaviors, hoping against hope there was some pill or innovative therapy.

"That's the Alzheimer's clinginess," he replied. "There's nothing you can do about that."

I turned to the Internet and found several articles that said the clinginess and following are common Alzheimer's behaviors.

"Unless his safety will be jeopardized, it's OK to let him follow you," one writer advised cheerfully.

That advice was useless and exasperating. What did she mean, *let him* follow me? I was seeking advice in the first place because I was powerless to stop him from following me or staring at me. If I walked into a burning building or off the edge of a cliff, he would be right behind me. Well, three feet behind me. No one seemed to care that an innocent woman was being driven insane in her own home.

I knew the clinging was preferable to the anger and violence some Alzheimer's patients exhibit. I knew that I was Gery's only anchor in a terrifying world. I knew that someday, there would be nothing I'd want more than to have him back at home, following me. I knew I was dealing with a child in the body of a man. Most of all, I knew the problem wasn't Gery's actions. The problem was my reaction.

I understood the situation intellectually, and I knew an expert in Alzheimer's behaviors could explain exactly why Gery was doing all these exasperating things. But there was no explanation that could help me tolerate the smothering clinginess I lived with each day.

I wish I could tell you that I learned to accept the following and the staring or that I developed a clever way to stop it. Though I adjusted to many other equally challenging behaviors, the clinginess was the nut I could never crack.

I told myself that Gery would stop following me and, eventually, he did. I guess there are times when your only option is to grit your teeth and carry on.▼

Remember. . . Not all behaviors last the duration of the illness.

progress? How many more times would I wipe urine off the bathroom floor, and what would I do when he became completely incontinent? Is this how I'd spend the rest of my life? These are the questions that haunted me. They may explain why caregivers get sick and why some die first.

The physical manifestations of bad stress are not subtle. I ground my teeth while I slept and cracked four of my teeth. I had chronic acid reflux. My neck muscles were so taut I sometimes had difficulty turning my head. I had headaches and chest pains. As the physical demands of caregiving increased, my osteoarthritis got worse.

During the six months before Gery went into long term care, I began having dizzy spells. I had one while we were driving on the highway, and I pulled over to the shoulder because I was afraid I would pass out at the wheel.

Experts recommend caregivers have at least four hours a week free from caregiving. Only twenty percent get that time.

All these symptoms were significantly reduced when I was no longer caring for Gery at home. For the first time in months, I was able to sleep a full night without interruption. People started telling me that I looked better. As I look back on my time as a caregiver, I wonder how I survived it. Sometimes I wonder if I have survived it.

I'm not an expert on the physiology or the psychology of stress, though it was my faithful companion throughout Gery's illness. More than one research study suggests that being a full-time caregiver for someone with Alzheimer's damages your immune system and can shorten your life by as much as eight years. This is why experts recommend that caregivers have at least four hours a week when they are completely free from caregiving. Unfortunately, only twenty percent of caregivers get that time.

The realistic option is finding small ways here and there to let air

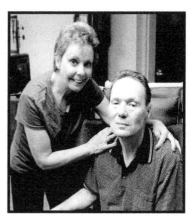

GERY'S 60TH BIRTHDAY, SIX MONTHS BEFORE HIS DEATH

out of your stress balloon. This might be the difference between surviving and drowning in a sea of cortisol.

Make no promises to yourself or anyone else about how long you'll be a caregiver. No one can predict the progression of the disease, how you will deal with the demands of caregiving over the long haul or how it might affect your health. For example, many people with Alzheimer's sleep twelve or more hours a day. Gery did the opposite. The more his disease progressed, the less he slept. When he was awake, I was awake, too. The lack of sleep finally forced me to throw in the towel. I never could have predicted this.

I tried to do one thing for myself every day, such as doing paper crafts for a half hour, walking around the block alone or cooking something special that I wanted for dinner.

Time alone was rare, so when someone took Gery on an outing, I never went along.

We bought a used hot tub and, after I got Gery to bed, I spent an hour blissfully soaking away the tension. Looking forward to my nocturnal dip often got me through the day. I had to remember to take my keys since Gery sometimes got up and locked the back door.

I was extremely fortunate to have a network of women friends who were an unwavering source of support and a sounding board for my sadness and angst. My children and their wonderful spouses were always there for me, and my grandchildren were a reliable source of joy. My family provided a reason to look forward to my future, though Gery wouldn't be part of it.

The most important thing I can tell you about surviving the stress is that there will be an end. You will have a life after caregiving. You won't comprehend that at first because it's impossible to see past the overwhelming challenges you're facing. But don't lose sight of the fact that there will be an end.

A friend advised me to think about how I would feel looking back on the experience of caregiving. It didn't take long to realize that I didn't want my post-caregiver years tainted by guilt and regret. No one could ever handle such a challenging situation perfectly, but I hoped I could say I'd done my best. Many times, I thought of my mother and grandmothers and the terrible hardships over which they triumphed. I like to think they are watching and are proud of me.

The following quote is from the National Organization for Empowering Caregivers. I wish I'd found it when I was a caregiver and I hope it will help you.

"Take a deep breath and acknowledge all that you are doing. You are an unsung hero. Embrace the beauty of who you are in this moment."▼

Remember. . . You will have a life after caregiving.

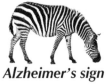

Alzheimer's sign

Gery's demeanor was passive and strangely absent. The young woman who cut our hair said, "Gery's a great guy, but it's like he isn't there."

Tears are not the mark of weakness, but of power. They are messengers of overwhelming grief and unspeakable love.

WASHINGTON IRVING
author and essayist

CHAPTER 19

Cry me a river

In the months after I learned my husband had Alzheimer's, crying became a staple in my daily routine. I was so sad that I could burst into tears at any moment of the day. I was afraid I might start crying and never stop. I was somewhat hampered because I didn't want Gery to see, but I got really good at finding opportunities to cry.

I cried in the shower. I cried in the car driving to the grocery store. I cried in the basement doing laundry. I cried running the vacuum cleaner. I cried shoveling snow and mowing the grass. I cried in public restrooms. I cried on the front stoop and on the back patio. I cried nearly every time someone asked me, "How is Gery doing?"

Many of my crying jags left me feeling limp and drained. The weeping was so frequent and so uncontrolled that it started to worry me. I wondered if all the crying was actually making me feel worse. I checked on the Internet and learned something interesting: no one has ever died from crying. The only way to die from crying would be to lose enough fluid to become fatally dehydrated. Even I couldn't cry that much.

The only way to die from crying would be to lose enough fluid to become fatally dehydrated. Even I couldn't cry that much.

I was encouraged by what I read. Mental health experts implied that people under long term toxic stress might be at risk from *not* crying. Humans laugh and cry instinctively, and we are the only creatures who cry as a result of emotions. Experts say people shed three types of tears. One type keeps our eyes lubricated, the second type is a reflex reaction to environmental irritants such as pollen or dust, and the last type is triggered by emotion. When scientists analyzed the content of the three tear types, they found something very interesting. While the first two types contain mostly water, emotional tears contain chemicals, including one that is associated with stress and another that helps to improve mood.

Though more study is needed, researchers theorize that stress hormones—the same hormones that have been proven to damage our bodies—are released when we cry. The Japanese have gotten serious about the potential benefits of crying. They've organized groups that regularly meet to watch sad movies and cry.

Remember. . . There is a reason they call it a "good" cry.

I stopped being concerned about how much I was crying. My complete inability to bottle up the terrible feelings was a blessing. During the first few years of my husband's illness, I cried a river of tears that washed away the poisonous emotions threatening my long term health and well-being.

If you feel like crying, it's unhealthy to hold it in. Have a good cry as often as you want. There is relief and release to be found in tears. They are a gift from God.▼

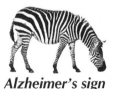

Alzheimer's sign

Gery came home one night and told me he had forgotten to turn off his car in the hospital parking lot. One of his colleagues came into the doctor's lounge and said, "Gery, do you know you left your car running?" He was very embarrassed and upset.

*Every evening I turn
my worries over to God.
He's going to be
up all night anyway.*

MARY CROWLEY
founder, Home Interiors
and Gifts

CHAPTER 20

Someone who is always there

People who don't believe in God or doubt God's existence sometimes point out that, despite the well-known saying, there have been plenty of atheists in fox holes. Ernest Hemingway is often cited as an example. I'm not sure if Hemingway was actually in a foxhole, but he was in the thick of several wars and lived to write classic (and lucrative) novels based on his experiences.

However, since Hemingway also shot himself in the head at age sixty-one because he couldn't face his declining health, I'm not sure he's a legitimate example of godless courage.

When Gery and I moved back to our hometown, we joined the First Presbyterian Church, Gery's childhood church. I had been raised in a church across town, but when we learned Gery was ill I was glad I let him choose our church. As the disease progressed, he was increasingly comforted by long-familiar people and places.

The atmosphere of warm and loving acceptance was a refuge in a world that didn't always show forbearance.

In the years to come, our church family was a blessing in our lives. We tried to contribute—we served as deacons and I joined the choir—but we got far more than we gave. I will be forever grateful for the emotional and spiritual support we received.

Gery was always happy when Sunday rolled around. I suspect the atmosphere of warm and loving acceptance was a refuge for him in a world that didn't always show forbearance to people with dementia. For me, attending church each Sunday brought a welcome sense of normalcy into our relentlessly abnormal world.

My dear friend Susan, whose husband is also in the choir, sat with Gery every Sunday during the service. As time passed, keeping him calm and in one place for an hour presented a challenge. Without her, I couldn't have sung in the choir, something that gave me joy at a time when joy was scarce.

Every Thursday, weather and schedules permitting, another wonderful church friend took Gery for a long walk in the park. For a stressed and weary caregiver, an hour or two alone was a gift more precious than gold. Shirley's kindness contributed greatly to my emotional well-being.

A month after Gery went to the nursing home, my pregnant daughter-in-law in Las Vegas was placed on complete bedrest. She needed help, so I flew out and stayed with them for three weeks. When I returned, our front steps, which had been falling apart for months, were magically repaired. I know my guardian angel was someone from the church. Though I asked repeatedly who had done it, no one would take the credit.

I was so terrified of what lay ahead that all pretense at eloquence deserted me. I shut my eyes, folded my hands and begged for help.

I was raised in a church-going family and attended parochial school through the eighth grade. However, as a young adult, I was focused on raising my children and furthering my career. Religious faith wasn't on my agenda or in my toolbox. I rarely went to church.

Then the man I love got a terminal illness and suddenly, I was the one in a foxhole. For the first time, I faced a challenge so daunting that I knew I couldn't handle it alone. In sheer desperation, I reached out for the Lord. I had pretty much ignored him for years, but he was still there.

I tried to pray, but I was so terrified of what lay ahead that all pretense at eloquence deserted me. Every Sunday, I shut my eyes, folded my hands and begged for help. "Please God, help me to be a better caregiver. Please God, give me the strength to deal with this."

During the first year Gery was ill, I had difficulty sleeping and frequently found myself wide awake at three a.m. While the rest of the world slept, I was awake wondering how I could live in this nightmare for one more minute. I've never felt so alone and frightened. I've never felt so humbled.

Again and again, I took refuge in my simple prayer, though I wondered if God wanted to hear from me. Eventually, I believed that he was listening. Some people say religious faith is a crutch, and they are absolutely right. But this crutch is a blessing, and I am glad to admit what a relief it was to put myself in God's hands.

Knowing Gery believed in heaven helped me face the final stage of his illness. I knew we would see each other again.

Every Sunday at the conclusion of the church service, our congregation recites the following charge: "Wherever we go, God has sent us. Wherever we are, God has put us there. He has a purpose in our being there. He has something he wants to do through us, wherever we are."

I taped this passage to our refrigerator, and I thought often about its meaning in my life. My wonderful friend Jane, who prayed faithfully for us throughout Gery's illness, was the first to suggest there was a divine purpose at work in our lives.

"Wherever we go, God has sent us." There was no satisfactory explanation for why bad things happen to good people, but I began to consider the possibility that there was a reason why Gery and I found each other again just a few years before he got sick.

"He has a purpose in our being there." What was God's purpose? At first I was impatient for answers, but in time I realized that the answers would come when I was ready to understand them. I suspect this process of spiritual growth and discovery will be a permanent part of my life journey.

CHAPTER 21

People will surprise you

When someone is dying—especially when someone is dying before their time—volatile emotions simmer close to the surface for everyone who loves the person. Relationships are tested. Some are strained beyond repair. The truly worthwhile ones get stronger.

As a caregiver for someone with a terminal illness, I was often surprised by how such an illness affects some people's behavior. I learned to abandon all my preconceived notions, because people won't always react as you think they will or should.

On the negative side is a phenomenon caregivers too often face. Don't be surprised if you and your decisions are criticized by people who didn't offer to help and have been blissfully uninvolved. You will be criticized by people who have no notion what it means to be a caregiver and no clue about the unimaginable challenges you've faced. The unfairness of it will make you angry and resentful.

Don't squander your emotional capital on eleventh hour critics. Avoid anyone who evokes negative feelings. If you foresee a situation in which you doubt your ability to hold your tongue, do yourself a huge favor and stay away.

A caregiver's emotional energy is a precious commodity. Don't waste it on other people's karma.

You can't change anyone's behavior, but the good news is you won't have to answer for it, either. A caregiver's emotional energy is a scarce commodity. Don't waste it on other people's karma.

Sometimes distant acquaintances and complete strangers say and do insensitive things.

About a year into Gery's illness, we went to the federal courthouse for a legal conference regarding his long term disability
benefits. Anxiety was a prominent Alzheimer's symptom for Gery,
and it was magnified tenfold in a situation like this one. When we
pased through the metal detector and the guard asked for our picture
IDs, Gery's hands shook so badly he couldn't even get his wallet out
of his pocket. As I tried to help him, a line formed behind us. A
second guard approached and asked, "What's going on here?" The
first guard said derisively, "This guy can't seem to find his ID."

I began to boil as Gery finally found his ID. I walked with him to
the stairs, asked him to wait for me and returned to where the guard
was sitting. "Hey, pal!" I said loudly. "My husband has Alzheimer's.
Think you could drum up a little sensitivity?" He looked shocked
and mumbled something as I stalked off.

I went into the restroom and was helping him unbuckle his pants when the door opened and I saw the flash of a camera.

At our 40-year class reunion about two months before Gery went
to the nursing home, there was a very unpleasant incident. Gery's
dementia was so severe that he had trouble with the basics of life. He
was surrounded by friends most of the evening, but when I saw him
head to the men's room, I followed. I knew he would need help, and
wanted to spare him embarrassment in front of our classmates.

I went into the restroom with him and was helping him unbuckle
his pants when the door opened and I saw the flash of a camera.
Clearly, someone thought something juicy was going on. When we
emerged from the restroom, I marched up to the photographer.
"Delete that picture!" I yelled.

Then there was the friend of a friend who told me that having to
put Gery in a nursing home shouldn't be a big deal since we had
been married just a few years. I was so stunned I was speechless.

One afternoon, I was sitting with Gery in the common room at the nursing home. A woman sat chatting with an elderly man, also a resident. Soon, one of the nurses came by. She had heard I was going to visit my son and his wife. "Have fun in Las Vegas!" she said.

The woman on the couch looked disapproving. "Oh, do you really think you should leave him?" she asked.

I felt as if I'd been slapped. "I'm not going out there to gamble. I'm going to see my grandsons," I choked. I pushed Gery's chair out of the room before I could say something I would regret.

No one was deliberately insensitive. In some situations, it's way too easy to say the wrong thing. But I hope these encounters taught people to think before speaking and to wait before judging strangers.

No one was deliberately insensitive. In some situations, it's way too easy to say the wrong thing.

The bad or disappointing behavior in some people is eclipsed by the people who surprise you in a good way.

Early in his illness, Gery flew to New York to visit his daughter. I didn't make the trip. I found a direct flight and got special permission to escort him to the gate. His daughter arranged to meet him at the gate in New York rather than in the terminal.

Even then, Gery became disoriented in strange surroundings. I took him to the gate and watched him disappear into the tunnel. I must have looked worried because when I turned to go, a woman in the passenger line stopped me and asked, "What's wrong with your husband, dear?" I told her he had Alzheimer's and that I was afraid he would get lost before his daughter saw him at the gate. She patted my hand reassuringly.

"Don't worry, I'll make sure he doesn't go off alone," she said.

My next door neighbor, who cared for her own husband for years before he died, was incredibly kind. Without being asked, she kept an eye on Gery while I was working. When Gery came outside, her grandson watched in case he wandered away.

I won't forget the kind young man from the local medical supply store who came twice to the nursing home to adjust Gery's CPAP mask. He refused to charge me despite the fact the machine didn't come from his store. The musicians who played at Gery's memorial refused to let me pay them, and told me to add the money to Gery's scholarship fund. When I went to the local print shop to get the programs for Gery's memorial, the owner refused to charge me.

Gery's best friend from childhood drove from two hours away every month to take Gery to lunch and visit him in the nursing home, though I know how much it hurt him to watch Gery deteriorate. My wonderful women friends were there for me without a second's hesitation whenever I asked for help. One of my friends even stayed all night with Gery so I could go to a college football game.

Gery's aunt welcomed him into her home when I had to attend meetings for my freelance business. Gery's sister called him every week and, after she retired, often drove over two hundred miles to spend the day with him. They will never know how Gery looked forward to these outings and how much their kindness meant to me.

My experience as a caregiver taught me to focus on the wonderful things so many people do. The bad things aren't always easy to leave behind, but that's where they belong.▼

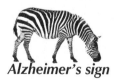

Alzheimer's sign

Gery's driving skills, never that good, seemed to deteriorate. We were driving in heavy traffic and Gery started to turn left in front of an oncoming semi. "I hope this guy can stop!" he announced gaily. Only my screams prevented a terrible accident.

*If I ever go looking
for my heart's desire
again, I won't look
further than my
own backyard.*

JUDY GARLAND AS DOROTHY
The Wizard of Oz

CHAPTER 22

Quietly memorable moments

The first thing many people do when they're diagnosed with a life-threatening illness is take a once-in-a-lifetime vacation. There's no more time for delayed gratification. It's now or never for that trip to Paris you've dreamed of for years or that cruise to Jamaica you postponed until retirement.

If your loved is mentally and physically capable of taking such a trip, I think it's a wonderful idea. If your loved one has Alzheimer's, take someone along to help you.

The most difficult experience for a person with Alzheimer's is being thrust into unfamiliar surroundings. The circumstance that led to Gery being diagnosed was our move to another state. Symptoms he was able to partially conceal in the familiar environs of his old medical practice roared to the surface in his new one. Within weeks of his arrival, everyone in the clinic knew something was wrong.

One of the most difficult experiences for someone with Alzheimer's is being thrust into unfamiliar surroundings.

About nine months after Gery was diagnosed, he went on a men-only fishing trip to Canada with Galen, the husband of one of my closest friends. Gery loved fishing and roughing it and really wanted to go. I had a premonition it had to be that summer or never. Galen has a mentally handicapped son and brother, so I trusted him implicitly with Gery's safekeeping. Away from me and our home, Gery was bound to become confused, but Galen didn't complain. I'll always be grateful to him. Gery told me he had a wonderful time.

Two years after his diagnosis, we flew to Las Vegas to visit my son and his wife, who had just had their first baby. Despite my joy over a new grandchild, Gery's dementia made for a difficult trip.

Just getting through the airport and onto the plane was incredibly stressful. Gery didn't know where he was supposed to go or what he was supposed to do. He walked three feet behind me wherever we went. He repeatedly left his suitcase behind.

At my son's house, Gery's anxiety was palpable. He refused to relax, pacing continually around the house. It put everyone on edge.

As a special treat for my birthday, my son got us tickets to the Cirque de Soleil Beatles show and made dinner reservations for us at the Mirage afterward. When we arrived at the restaurant, Gery went into the men's room while I waited by the hostess stand. When he didn't emerge after a reasonable time, I noticed that the restroom entrance and exit were separate, and that the exit was near the main casino walkway packed with hundreds of people on their way to various clubs. On the other side of the walkway was a door that led directly outside to the Las Vegas Strip.

I had hideous visions of Gery wandering down Las Vegas Boulevard—lost, frightened and confused.

A man came out of the restroom and I asked him if he noticed a tall thin man wearing a navy blue polo shirt in the restroom. "I was the only guy in there," he replied.

I had never been afraid of Gery getting lost in our hometown, but lost in Las Vegas was an entirely different matter. It's not likely that anyone will kidnap a fifty-eight-year-old dementia patient, but I had hideous visions of Gery wandering down Las Vegas Boulevard—lost, frightened and confused. Or worse, that he would be assaulted and robbed.

I went to the seating hostess and told her my husband had gotten lost coming out of the restroom and that he had Alzheimer's. I began to cry, and she put her arm around me. "Don't worry," she said. "We have cameras everywhere! We'll find him."

I gave her a description of Gery and she called hotel security. Twenty minutes later, a man I assumed was a plainclothes security guard appeared with Gery in tow. Gery came toward me with his arms outstretched.

"I'm sorry, sweetheart!" he exclaimed. I was so glad to see him that I forgot to ask where he'd gone. Gery hugged me and later I realized that he was the one comforting me, though he was the one who had gotten lost.

Despite the rocky start, we enjoyed our dinner. We were having coffee when Gery stood up and announced he was going to the restroom. A few feet away, a Hispanic busboy was clearing a table.

"Where he going now?" he asked in heavily accented English. "Do not lose him again!" Apparently, the story of the lost man had spread to the restaurant staff. I couldn't help but smile.

I had to accept that his dementia was too advanced for this kind of travel unless someone was along to help me.

Except for the Beatles show, Gery didn't enjoy the trip. I had to accept that his dementia was too advanced for this kind of travel unless someone was along to help me.

Later, I learned the hard way that Alzheimer's patients can't deal with chaos. We were celebrating our grandson's first birthday. Our small house was packed with people, many of whom Gery didn't know, and there was lots of commotion. I found Gery sitting on the couch, tears in his eyes. "All these people!" he whispered in anguish. "I don't know who any of them are!"

It was Saturday, and my friends were making the rounds of local garage sales. I called, they came and took Gery to lunch. They told me later that it took all three of them to keep him calm.

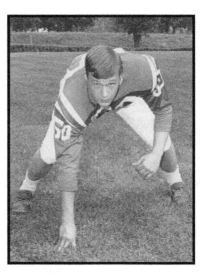

**GERY'S TEAM
PHOTO, 1967**

What I learned is that the very best memories were made with familiar people in familiar places. Our social life was confined to spending time with family and close friends, and Gery was never happier than when we were invited to someone's house for dinner or his sisters came for a barbeque. These moments weren't exiting or glamorous, but they were the most enjoyable for Gery.

The most memorable event by far during Gery's three years at home was a reunion of our high school football team. The fall of 2008 was the fortieth anniversary of the team from our senior year that won the conference championship. In a small town, this is big stuff. Gery was the starting center on the team. He suggested planning a reunion for the team at the homecoming game, and I thought it was a wonderful idea.

Our house is two blocks from the football field and the yard is well-suited to a large tailgate party. We mailed flyers to all the players, coaches and cheerleaders. We arranged for the team to be introduced during halftime of the football game. I designed a poster of team photos and records and, with mock solemnity, Gery said, "Honey, you've documented our greatness."

I was amazed by the turnout for the reunion. All but a handful of team members came, many from out of state. One of Gery's friends brought game films that were taken by his father. Late in the evening, someone tacked a sheet over our garage door, and we watched grainy black and white movies taken with the primitive 1960s-era camera.

Gery's long-term memory was still intact then, and he recalled every detail of the nine games he played our senior year. I can still see his handsome face as it looked in the flickering light. I can still hear him laughing and reminiscing with his teammates, the boys who became men together on the football field.

Many of our classmates said later that they'll never forget the reunion of the 1968 team. It is a bittersweet memory for me because of our shared awareness of Gery's illness and its implications for his future. I knew there was very little chance Gery would be planning a fiftieth reunion of his beloved Toreadors.

Gery's reunion was the perfect idea at the perfect time. It required a fair amount of work, but I will always be very glad we did it. It was by far the happiest time we enjoyed during his illness, and it happened right in our own backyard.▼

Remember. . . For someone with
Alzheimer's, there's no place like home.

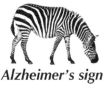

Alzheimer's sign

About nine months before we moved back to our hometown, we sold our house and moved into an apartment. Gery repeatedly asked me our new address and phone number.

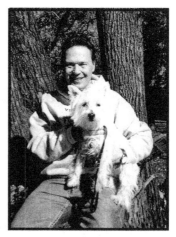

GERY AND LUCY, 2009

really predict who was going to die next, or if she was just looking for a warm place to nap.

But I know what I saw, and I believe Lucy knew that Gery had changed in some fundamental way. Whether she smelled it or saw it or heard it or sensed it, she knew something dogs aren't supposed to know. She may have known something I didn't know.

Despite their size and appearance, Westies are not lap dogs. Yet, as Gery's dementia progressed, Lucy took up permanent residence beside him on the couch. No matter what odd hour Gery decided to go to bed, Lucy went along. She lay next to him rather than at the foot of the bed, her preferred spot before Gery got sick.

Gery took Lucy on countless walks, sometimes five or six a day. My neighbor watched out her window because she was afraid Gery would get lost, and she swore to me that Lucy brought Gery back home, not the other way around.

Late in Gery's illness, everything changed again. I was making the bed one day and heard Gery in the living room talking to Lucy. He said her name several times. When I came out of the bedroom, I saw that Lucy wasn't in the living room. She was in the doorway watching Gery intently. Her little body was completely still and she tilted her head back and forth in that cute way dogs have of showing confusion. I went to the doorway and saw that Gery was talking to a pillow with an embroidered picture of a Westie.

For me, this was just one of many make-you-laugh, make-you-cry Alzheimer's moments, but I believe it was more than that for Lucy. Gery had crossed a line that was significant in the dog world. From that day on, her behavior changed. She stopped sitting by him and refused to lie beside him in bed. She acted almost as if she was afraid of him. Gery's dementia was so advanced that he didn't appear to notice.

From puppyhood, Lucy was a moody dog, but when I placed Gery in long-term care, her behavior became downright neurotic. She disappeared for long periods and I found her in weird places—in a closet, beneath a table, in a corner of the basement or behind the toilet. Sometimes she followed me when I left the room. When she wasn't hiding, she was staring at me anxiously. The vet said Lucy was in mourning and, like human grief, there is no specific timetable for how long it will last.

I took Lucy to visit Gery in the nursing home. He was in a recliner in the hallway. When he saw her, his mouth formed a huge "O" of surprise and he flapped his arms in delight. It was by far the biggest reaction Gery exhibited for any visitor to the nursing home.

Though Lucy sat beside Gery in his chair, she was visibly uncomfortable. I took her back for a second visit, but Gery didn't react to her at all, and Lucy was terrified. She hid under my chair, shaking, and I had to drag her out. Clearly, she didn't like this place.

That was her last visit. She had already done so much for Gery and I couldn't ask more of her.▼

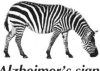

Alzheimer's sign

Gery bought a sidewalk edger but couldn't figure out how it worked. He gave up, put it in the garage and never tried to use it again.

*Try to surround them with
many familiar things
so they maintain
a sense of security.*

CAROL ROACH
*Ways of Dealing with
Alzheimer's Behaviors*

CHAPTER 24

I simply remember my favorite things

Years ago, a friend told me that her four-year-old daughter would have happily watched the movie "Bedknobs and Broomsticks" at least five times a day. I thought of this as Gery's illness progressed and he became more and more childlike in his preference for all things familiar.

When Gery could no longer work and didn't seem to know how to entertain himself, I tried unsuccessfully to interest him in a variety of movies, books, television shows and foods. I couldn't believe he really was content with such a limited menu of life's possibilities. Finally, I put aside my ideas about what constitutes enjoyable entertainment or a good meal and began paying closer attention to what made Gery happy.

I decided it was better to serve only his favorite foods, even if I got bored with the severely limited menu.

He'd always loved my cooking and ate anything I put in front of him. However, as the disease progressed, he was not enthused about most foods. If I gave him something new, or something that wasn't one of his favorites, he was more likely to push his plate away half-eaten. When he began losing weight during his last months at home, I tried giving him a nutritional drink, but he said he didn't like it and refused to drink it. I decided it was better to serve only his favorite foods, even if I got bored with the severely limited menu.

For breakfast, he had homemade oatmeal. For lunch, a hamburger or a turkey sandwich with potato salad made by the local grocery store. Dinner was ham balls or meat loaf and fried potatoes, tuna casserole and corn muffins or chicken and pasta. Each night before bed, a dish of mint chocolate chip ice cream.

Gery had been on cholesterol medication since before we were married and was always conscious of his fat intake. During the diagnostic process, one of his doctors banned caffeine and alcohol from his diet. The day after we found out he had Alzheimer's, Gery announced that he would never again consume decaffeinated coffee, low-fat ice cream or faux beer. Nothing trumped Gery's comfort and happiness, so I bought regular coffee, real beer and full-fat ice cream.

During his final months at home, Gery watched the same four movies incessantly: John Wayne's classic "Sands of Iwo Jima", a movie about Winston Churchill called "Into the Storm", "Second-hand Lions" and—his absolute favorite—"The Blues Brothers."

His favorite "Blues Brothers" quote was "It's 106 miles to Chicago, we've got a full tank of gas, a half a pack of cigarettes, it's dark and we're wearing sunglasses." No matter how many times he'd watched the movie that week, he laughed heartily at that line.

Though Gery had always loved to read, there was only one book he picked up after he was diagnosed with Alzheimer's—a book about his father's World War II bomber group. I was astounded at how often each day he leafed through the pages of that book. I finally put a tray table next to the couch and placed the book there permanently.

Familiar things in familiar places are the only anchor in the upside-down world of Alzheimer's. How many times each week should someone watch the same movie, wear the same shirt, read the same book or eat the same foods? As many times as he wants.▼

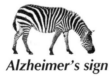

Alzheimer's sign

The air conditioning in Gery's car wouldn't work properly because he never pushed the button that recirculated air. I explained it to him several times, but he couldn't seem to remember.

I was at the pinnacle of my career one day, and the next day I was put out to pasture. I felt like a racehorse with a broken leg.

JACK KLUGMAN
actor diagnosed with
throat cancer

CHAPTER 25

Give him a job, any job

One day, not long after Gery was diagnosed, I came into the living room and saw him on the couch, his shoulders and face sagging.

"I feel useless," he said.

This was the first and last time I heard Gery say anything that sounded even remotely self-pitying. I felt useless, too, because I had no idea how to help him.

Gery was a notoriously hard worker. He prided himself on being one of the top producers in his seventy-physician primary care group. He boasted that he had never missed a day of work because of illness. The work ethic in his family was very strong. His father and his aunt, both doctors, practiced into their eighties.

When Alzheimer's forced him into early retirement at age fifty-six, he was completely and utterly lost.

When Gery and I were first married, several of his coworkers and friends told me they were concerned that Gery was literally working himself to death. They hoped I could convince him to slow down. I enjoyed modest success. I acquainted him with the novel concept of relaxing at home by buying him a pair of sweatpants and insisting that he change out of his work clothes for a few hours each night. I started talking with him about what we would do when we retired. At my urging, he began taking an occasional afternoon off. I kept him from going to work the day his brother died.

However, sixty-hour work weeks were still the rule rather than the exception. When Alzheimer's forced him into early retirement at age fifty-six, he was completely and utterly lost. He had no hobbies. He

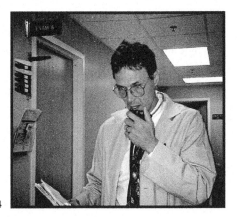

GERY IN HIS CLINIC, 1994

had no initiative to start new projects, and he wasn't interested in reading or any other sedentary pursuit. His only desire was to help me, and he counted on me to tell him how to do it.

One of my greatest challenges during Gery's illness was dealing with his burning desire to help me around the house when he wasn't really capable of it.

It wasn't difficult at first. I typed step-by-step instructions on how to run the dishwasher, dryer, etc. and taped them prominently on each appliance. Every day before I left for work, I gave Gery a 'to do' list containing at least five tasks. Coming up with tasks I thought he could handle wasn't always easy, but I did fairly well.

He was really good at cleaning the top of my gas stove, and he actually seemed to enjoy it. That task was on Gery's list so often that we had the cleanest stove top in town. He was also very good at sweeping the wooden floors, something that could be done each day. Gery checked off each task as he completed it and, like a child seeking praise, showed me the list when I got home from work.

Within a year of his diagnosis, things disintegrated. Gery was still obsessed with helping me around the house and got upset if I told him there was nothing for him to do, but he could no longer follow the simplest instructions or remember anything I said.

Every day, he took dirty dishes out of the dishwasher and put them in the cupboards. He took dirty clothes out of the hamper and put them into the dressers. When I carried groceries into the house, he carried them back out to the car when I wasn't looking.

There were days when he asked "How can I help you?" so many times it was surreal. Each time he asked, his tone was increasingly aggressive. One day, after hearing the question at least ten times, I suggested in complete desperation that he gather sticks. We have large trees and the yard is always full of sticks, so what could be better? What task could be simpler? I was proud of my ingenuity.

Seconds later, he was back in the house, claiming he couldn't find any sticks. "How can I help you?" he demanded again. I had to leave the room to keep from screaming in frustration.

Every two weeks I cleaned our house, mostly to preserve some sense of normalcy. Gery liked cleaning day and insisted on helping. It was his job to get the vacuum cleaner from the basement. As his dementia worsened, he wasn't able to complete even that simple task. He went to the basement twice and, both times, returned empty-handed. I went to get it myself and, of course, he followed me. When I picked up the vacuum, he exclaimed, "Let me do that!" and angrily jerked it out of my hand.

By the time cleaning day mercifully ended, my chest ached and my head pounded from the stress caused by Gery's attempts to help.

By the time cleaning day mercifully ended, my head pounded from the stress of dealing with Gery's attempts to help.

Lawn mowing day was equally challenging. Gery thought lawn care was his job, but I was afraid to let him use the mower. Visibly angry, he stalked along beside me as I pushed the mower back and forth. "Let me do it!" he yelled, becoming increasingly agitated. I tried to ignore him, or told him he could mow later. No matter what I said, he continued to follow me. Sometimes I cried from pure frustration. I imagine these events were interesting for our neighbors. Every Monday, Gery went to an adult day care center for a few hours. I was advised to use that time to do something fun. When I had an outside job, I worked while he was there. When I had to quit my job, I often used the time to mow the lawn or clean the house. I was in survival mode, and my new idea of fun was cleaning and mowing without Gery.

The light finally came on in the spring of 2010, about six months before Gery went to the nursing home. It was late afternoon and, as usual, Gery exhibited growing anxiety. His hands trembled and he sighed repeatedly. He jumped up from the couch every few minutes and paced. It had already been a long day and I knew it would be a longer night. I hoped some fresh air might calm him down.

"Gery!" I said loudly. "I need your help." He stopped pacing and looked at me. "I really need your help," I repeated. "Please go out and check the tomato plants. I'm worried they're not OK."

Throughout the spring and summer, I repeatedly sent Gery and Lucy into the back yard on hilariously pointless errands.

He looked interested and asked if Lucy could go along. I put the dog on her leash and they went outside. I looked out the bedroom window every few minutes to make sure he hadn't wandered off, though I knew Lucy would bring him back if he did.

He was outside for nearly twenty minutes before he came back into the house and told me the tomato plants looked good. I praised him lavishly for helping me. He beamed with pleasure.

Throughout the spring and summer, I repeatedly sent Gery and Lucy into the back yard on hilariously pointless errands. I asked him to check the tomato plants. I asked him to count the tomato plants. When the vines began to bear fruit, I asked him to count the growing tomatoes. He particularly liked this assignment.

CHAPTER 26

What do you think you are, a saint?

> ### PERFECT CAREGIVER WANTED
>
> *Qualified candidates possess endless patience, unflagging energy, unshakable courage and sunny good humor despite toxic stress and daily frustration. Must be physically fit, dexterous, constantly vigilant, gently sympathetic and able to operate at peak efficiency on very little sleep. No sick leave, no vacations, extremely limited time off, 168 hours per week.*

There was nothing saintly in my caregiving and I fell far short of the paragon described in this fictional want ad. I got impatient with Gery and sometimes it showed. I tried hard not to snap at him, but I didn't always succeed. I tried hard to keep him from seeing my despair, but there were times when I failed miserably.

After every lapse, I punished myself severely. What kind of a self-absorbed person can't control her mood swings for the sake of her dying spouse? What kind of a terrible person gets irritated with someone who has a terminal illness? Every time I lost my patience or my poker face, I hated myself. Every time, I told myself it would never happen again. Every time, I went into another room and silently mouthed these words: *He can't help it. He's doing his best.*

Looking back, it's so obvious what I was missing. The mantra I repeated over and over to myself? It also applied to me! I couldn't help it either! Like Gery, I was doing my best.

We aren't saints. We're mortals who have been thrust by fate into an awful situation. When a terrible disease happens to someone in your family, it happens to you, too. Give yourself a break. Stop holding yourself to impossible standards.▼

Crying is all right,
but sooner or later
you have to stop, and
then you still have to
decide what to do.

CS LEWIS
Irish writer and scholar

CHAPTER 27

Delaying the inevitable

During the summer and fall of 2010 when I was struggling to accept that it was time to put Gery in long-term care, I was told the following three stories:

A woman cared for her elderly parents in their home. Her father had diabetes, her mother had Alzheimer's. Before he died, her father made her promise she would never take her mother to a nursing home. After several years of caring for her mother, she couldn't handle it anymore and placed her in a care facility. Every time she visited, she was overwhelmed by guilt.

A man was determined that his father, who had Alzheimer's, would never go to a nursing home. He cared for him at home for years and was hailed as a saint by everyone who knew him. Then it was discovered that every day, in sheer desperation, he tied his father to a chair in the basement.

A man with early onset Alzheimer's was cared for at home by his wife. When caregiving became too difficult, she decided to admit him to a nursing home. She was severely criticized by her sister-in-law, who told everyone she was dumping her brother at a nursing home so she could be fancy free. The critical sister brought her brother to her house, where she cared for him for three days before resigning from the job.

Recently, my daughter told me that in the months before Gery went to the nursing home, she and her brother were so concerned about my well-being they were planning to intervene in the hope of convincing me that I couldn't continue caring for him at home.

Early in Gery's illness, I seriously considered keeping him at home until the end. I was by no means confident I'd be able to do it, but the alternative seemed unthinkable. I just couldn't face the prospect of putting Gery in a nursing home when he was so young. I discussed it with my friends, who were less than enthusiastic. I talked to my sister-in-law, who'd cared for Gery's brother for eighteen months, through his liver failure, transplant and death at home. She was adamant that I shouldn't try to keep Gery at home until he died. She knew we couldn't afford full time help, and she said I wouldn't be able to handle the physical demands of caring for someone in the final stage of Alzheimer's. She had been a caregiver, and she'd had a long career as a surgical nurse. If she said I couldn't do it, I saw no reasonable course but to accept her judgment.

Within a year of his diagnosis, Gery was well into stage four. One of his doctors urged me to start looking into long-term care.

I've always been grateful we had that conversation. I may have come to the same conclusion on my own eventually, but now I had time to accept the idea that, in all likelihood, I would be forced to take Gery to a long-term care facility.

A few weeks after his diagnosis, Gery raised the issue of who would care for him as the disease progressed. His tone was typically matter-of-fact. "Don't try to take care of me at home," he cautioned. "Take me to a nursing home right away."

His words shocked me, and I chose my answer carefully. "I'll do it as long as I can," I replied.

He seemed satisfied with my answer and we never discussed it again. When I consider the selfless courage behind his admonition, I am amazed all over again by the man I married.

Experts have divided the progression of Alzheimer's into seven stages. Within a year of his diagnosis, Gery was well into stage four and one of his doctors urged me to start investigating long-term care options. I was surprised to hear the subject mentioned so soon. Caring for him was getting more difficult, but I wasn't ready for this.

I thought about what the doctor said and decided I would consider long-term care when Gery no longer recognized me. Back then, I didn't understand that not recognizing someone and not being able to produce that person's name would not be the same thing for Gery.

Eighteen months later, Gery still recognized me most of the time but the burden of his care was getting heavier by the day. He gave a deceptively normal impression in casual and brief encounters, but his behavior at home was increasingly difficult to deal with. His mobility and his advanced dementia were a dangerous combination, and I couldn't let him out of my sight. Once again, I was the mother of a toddler. Only this toddler would never grow up, and I was no longer young.

Once again, I was the mother of a toddler. Only this toddler would never grow up and I was no longer young.

He did things that jeopardized his health and safety, such as eating raw beef from the refrigerator and opening the car door while the car was moving. He could no longer dress himself, take a shower or go to the bathroom alone. He slept less and less at night and never napped during the day. I called his neurologist and we tried several medications to help him sleep. No medication worked the way it was supposed to. A side effect of one of the drugs was the urge to urinate, which made Gery wake up more often.

After the third medication failed, the neurologist told me there was nothing left to try. He strongly recommended that I place Gery in long term care before my health was permanently affected.

I toured a local nursing home. It was a nice place, but it made me so sad I wanted to run away to avoid the terrible decision looming in my immediate future. I continued to drag my feet and several weeks passed before I completed the paperwork and Gery's name was placed on a waiting list.

His last weeks at home were awful, especially the nights. His sleep disturbances continued, and occasionally he was incontinent. Several times, I caught him leaving the house at two or three a.m. I have no idea how he was able to unlock the door. I hadn't been well-rested for several years, and now I was exhausted. As much as I dreaded taking Gery to the nursing home, I knew I couldn't face the demands of caregiving every day with so little sleep.

The nursing home director called and said a room was available, but I declined. She called again in a couple of weeks and I knew I couldn't delay the inevitable any longer. I took Gery to his new home on a sunny Saturday in October of 2010, almost three years to the day after he was diagnosed.

A change in environment is extremely traumatic for people with Alzheimer's, and Gery's transition was just as difficult as I feared it would be. He believed he was there to make nursing home rounds, and he was awake for seventy-two straight hours. His eyes were bloodshot; his movements seemed frantic. He gave no indication he even saw me when I went to visit him. When I saw the state he was in, I felt ill. I left as quickly as I could and sat in my car crying. It took nearly a month before he began to adjust.

A change in environment is traumatic for people with Alzheimer's. Gery's transition was just as difficult as I feared it would be.

The first week he was gone, I went to bed at nine each night and slept the clock around. I've never slept so much. Within weeks, nearly all of the physical manifestations of stress I had experienced for three years were significantly reduced.

A nurse who took care of Gery told me the staff couldn't imagine how I'd cared for him without a live-in nurse. When I called Gery's closest friends to tell them he was in a nursing home, several of them thanked me for taking care of him at home for so long. It was very reassuring to hear this from people who truly loved Gery.

No one criticized my decision, at least not to my face. It wouldn't have mattered anyway. From my perspective, several things were obvious. It's easy to criticize a decision to place someone in long-term care if you aren't the one doing the caregiving. It's just as easy to advise putting someone in long-term care when it's not your relative who won't get to live at home and will be cared for by strangers.

From the beginning, I knew this would be the most difficult decision I'd ever have to make. Taking him to a nursing home was the end of our life together, and it felt like the end of our marriage, too. Leaving my sweetheart behind and walking away tore a hole in my heart, but the decision had to be mine and no one else's. I had to own it because I would live with it for the rest of my life.

The passage of time often brings things into focus. I know that I probably waited six months too long to place him, but I'd much rather live with that than wonder if I could have kept him at home for a few more months or even a few more weeks. He was my husband, he was too young for a nursing home and things had to get really, really bad before I could bring myself to do it.

I fulfilled the promise I made to Gery and to myself. I did it as long as I could.▼

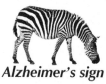

Alzheimer's sign

Doctors must be re-certified in their specialties every ten years. Gery jokingly told me, "If I ever score less than ninety percent on the family practice boards, you'll know something is wrong with me." When I was going through his memorabilia after he died, I found his test from 1980, the first time he took the boards. He scored ninety-nine percent. I also found his test results from July of 2006, which I had never seen. His score was fifty-nine percent.

I heard someone whisper,
'My father has Alzheimer's.'
I said, 'You don't
have to whisper,
shout it out loud!

PARTICIPANT IN AN
ALZHEIMER'S ASSOCIATION
TOWN MEETING

CHAPTER 28

The disease of denial

Gery had been in the nursing home for two months when, in one of life's little ironies, my ninety-six year-old aunt moved into the room across the hall. Sitting with us near the nurses' station one day, she looked at Gery and asked, "When did he go crazy?"

My aunt was suffering from dementia (though not as severe as Gery's) and she was known for her frankness. But her question revealed an attitude that is secretly held by many people. There are many unpleasant surprises that accompany an Alzheimer's diagnosis. For me, one of the most unpleasant was the discovery that there is a very real stigma against this disease.

In 1994 when Ronald Reagan announced he had Alzheimer's, he was praised by the head of the Alzheimer's Association, who said President Reagan's openness would dispel the stigma against the disease. Nearly twenty years later, there is still much to be done to make this statement a reality.

It's ludicrous to be ashamed of a pathological process simply because it occurs in the brain rather than in the heart or lungs.

I first learned of the stigma through my freelance work for the Iowa Association of County Medical Examiners. A woman with the Iowa Bureau of Vital Records told me people frequently demand that 'dementia' be listed as their relative's cause of death rather than Alzheimer's. This information was confirmed by several forensic pathologists, who told me that literally no one wants Alzheimer's recorded as the cause of death on a relative's death certificate.

Alzheimer's is a disease. It occurs at the cellular level and can be seen on an MRI or PET scan or at autopsy. It is ludicrous to be ashamed of a pathological process simply because it occurs in the brain rather than in the heart or lungs. An Iowa doctor who specializes in end-of-life care said, "Modern medicine has defined heart failure. kidney failure and liver failure. It's time to define brain failure."

Many advocates predict that the number of people with Alzheimer's will double by 2025. It's only a matter of time before everyone knows someone with Alzheimer's. Perhaps a greater understanding of this disease will free it from the stigma.

When Gery was diagnosed, I asked him how he felt about people finding out he had Alzheimer's. He said, "I'm not embarrassed." Like Ronald Reagan, Charlton Heston, Glen Campbell and Tennessee women's basketball coach Pat Summitt, Gery had the courage to be open and honest.

If we truly want to make a difference for future Alzheimer's patients, we must start in our own little worlds. From the day Gery was diagnosed, we refused to behave as though this was something to be ashamed of and concealed.

Many of today's obituaries list no cause of death. Gery's obituary stated without equivocation that he died from complications of early onset Alzheimer's. On his death certificate, Alzheimer's is recorded as the cause of death.

Death certificates are an important source of information for policy makers who decide where research dollars will be spent. I want Gery to be counted.▼

Remember. . . Alzheimer's is a disease, not a mental illness.

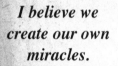

*I believe we
create our own
miracles.*

MICHAEL LANDON
actor who died of
pancreatic cancer

CHAPTER 29

Our contribution to the search

Shortly after a neurologist at the Mayo Clinic confirmed Gery's diagnosis, we enrolled in the trial of a new Alzheimer's drug. For the next two years, we traveled to Mayo—a seven-hour round trip— every six weeks. The visits consisted of either intravenous doses of the drug or a battery of tests.

I'm glad we did it. An effective treatment will never be found if people don't participate in research, especially people like Gery who are otherwise healthy.

On a personal level, the drug study offered a glimmer of hope at a time when hope was nearly impossible to come by. Even the remotest chance that the drug might ease the symptoms sustained me as I struggled to accept the reality of Gery's illness. Gery was motivated by a desire to help others, and by my desire to participate. He didn't believe in medical miracles.

Gery was motivated by a desire to help others, and by my desire to participate. He didn't believe in medical miracles.

In conjunction with the drug trial, Gery got some fairly exotic blood tests which we could never have afforded on our own. As a result of these tests, we learned that Gery is a carrier of a blood protein called e4 allele that greatly increases one's risk of Alzheimer's. The neurologist told us this protein is inherited, valuable information for Gery's blood relatives.

We fell into a routine for the trips and, though he generally didn't do well away from home, Gery became comfortable with it. We always drove up the day before the appointment, stayed in the same hotel and ate at the same restaurant. We spent our afternoons browsing the shelves at Barnes & Noble. Though the reason for the traveling was far from pleasant, I look back fondly on those trips. I feel satisfied we did all we could to make them enjoyable.

On the debit side, enrolling in a drug trial affected my potential employment. I didn't have a job when Gery was diagnosed because we had just relocated. I got a part time job so that I could travel to the Mayo Clinic every six weeks. However, I was forced to quit that job a year later anyway because Gery couldn't be left alone.

There was a negative aspect for Gery. The mental status testing caused him increasing anxiety. One of the testers told me she had never seen anyone try so hard. As his brain function deteriorated, so did his test performance. He knew he was doing poorly and that it was undeniable evidence of the disease.

When Gery was tested during our final Mayo visit, he was unable to identify a stethoscope. He was so distraught he couldn't sleep that night. Despite his advancing dementia and severely impaired short term memory, several days passed before he forgot about it.

Sometimes I think it would have been better for him to remain blissfully ignorant of how far the Alzheimer's had progressed in such a short time.

This was our experience; yours may be completely different. Participating in a clinical trial is a significant commitment and there is no right or wrong answer. It's a decision only you can make, based on your circumstances and feelings.▼

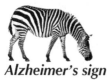

Alzheimer's sign

I went to visit friends out of state and when I returned, the mailbox was so full the door wouldn't close. Gery hadn't gotten the mail the entire time I was gone.

There is something fascinating about science. One gets such wholesale returns of conjecture out of such a trifling investment of fact.

MARK TWAIN
Life on the Mississippi

CHAPTER 30

Medical news and healthy skepticism

Because so many Alzheimer's questions remain unanswered, there is a virtual sea of myths, misconceptions and misinformation about the disease. The cavernous knowledge gap makes Alzheimer's an attractive target for purveyors of junk science.

Here is just a sampling of the Alzheimer's myths that populate the Internet:

• Silver dental fillings can cause Alzheimer's.
• The artificial sweetener aspartame can lead to Alzheimer's.
• Dietary supplements can protect your brain from Alzheimer's.
• Exposure to aluminum can cause Alzheimer's.
• Flu shots can increase your risk of Alzheimer's.
• Anti-inflammatory drugs can slow Alzheimer's dementia.

Here's one I latched onto: playing intellectually challenging games can slow the progression of Alzheimer's. Early in Gery's illness, I read this on several websites and believed it. I must have been temporarily insane. The progression of Gery's dementia was rapid and relentless. It's ludicrous to assert that thinking of words and numbers in a puzzle could restrain such an inexorable process.

The cavernous knowledge gap makes Alzheimer's an attractive target for purveyors of junk science.

Back then, I was still struggling to get used to the idea that Gery had Alzheimer's. I was vulnerable and desperate to do something to help, so I bought books of crossword and sudoku puzzles and tried to get him to do them. There was just one problem—Gery wasn't interested. Though doctors had advised him to keep his mind active, he didn't once pick up a puzzle book on his own. He was very happy to do a puzzle if I sat beside him and supplied all the answers. These sessions invariably ended with Gery looking anxious and me feeling exasperated. Not only did this not help, it made the situation worse. Maybe this was evidence of a common early symptom of Alzheimer's—lack of initiative. Maybe he knew he wasn't capable of doing crossword puzzles or playing computerized chess even then. Maybe his attention span was more compromised than I realized. Gery was so affably non-compliant that it was difficult to judge. I believe he was humoring me.

Looking back, I wonder if he knew there was nothing to be gained except a sense of acute frustration for both of us. Gery had an uncanny ability to avoid situations that called attention to his illness. In that, he was much wiser than his caregiver.

In most cases, no harm will come from trying the new theories. I fully understand that there are people who want to test every new idea involving foods or spices or vitamins that may arrest or prevent Alzheimer's. Gery wasn't among them.

I wish the media would do a better job of scrutinizing the science before they present news of so-called breakthroughs. My husband's time was precious and no one had a right to waste it.▼

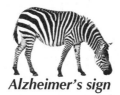

Alzheimer's sign

The application for an Iowa medical license asks about any criminal history. When Gery was filling it out, he became fixated on a night in 1972 when he and two friends were stopped by police. Gery wasn't driving, but was celebrating his twenty-first birthday with multiple beers and loud singing. He was charged with disturbing the peace. He revised his written description of this crime spree numerous times. At first, I thought he was joking.

The only thing
you take with you
when you're gone
is what you
leave behind.

JOHN ALLSTON
former president of
General Foods

CHAPTER 31

Picking up the pieces

In 2001, a few months before Gery and I got married, we had a serious disagreement about a serious subject—organ donation. Gery's younger brother Stan was desperately ill with a failing liver and Gery told me he planned to donate part of his liver to his brother. I was horrified.

Gery had lost his youngest brother to a seizure disorder in 1996, and I knew he was having difficulty facing Stan's illness. I also knew his decision to donate was emotional and not rooted in sound science. Liver transplants involving live donors were extremely experimental. Some transplant surgeons refused to do them. Several prestigious hospitals suspended live donor liver transplants when donors died after the surgery.

I presented the facts calmly and begged him to reconsider. He agreed, very reluctantly. Stan eventually got a donor liver from an accident victim.

When Gery went into hospice care, I asked the staff about organ donation. Organ donation was very important to Gery.

A year later, Stan's kidneys began to fail and Gery promised to donate one of his. Though I felt the gesture was futile, I knew that live donor kidney transplants are done successfully every day. I could think of no logical reason to object, and I could sense he wouldn't be dissuaded this time. Gery remained firm in his intention, despite a barrage of objections from other family members. Stan died before the surgery could be done.

When Gery went into hospice care, I asked the staff about organ

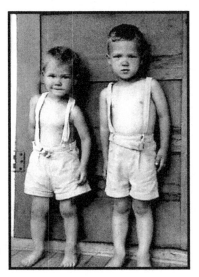

GERY (RIGHT) AND HIS BROTHER STAN, 1955

donation. I told them Gery was a strong proponent, and had even registered as an organ donor on the ID card he received in place of a driver's license.

In a few days, a hospice social worker told me Gery wouldn't qualify to be a donor. I was crushed. I felt that if Gery could help other people go on living, or improve the quality of someone's life, some good could come from this terrible situation. I asked why he couldn't donate; she didn't know.

I called the director of hospice. She was very kind, and her explanation made sense. People who donate organs have typically been in some kind of accident that requires them to be placed on life support. Throughout the process that leads to a declaration of brain death, a machine pumps blood through their bodies, keeping their organs alive and viable. Gery had a do-not-resuscitate order and would not die in the right way.

I asked whether Gery's do-not-resuscitate order would prevent him from donating his corneas, optic nerves and tissue. She didn't know the answer to that question, so she gave me the number of the Iowa Donor Network.

I spoke with the head of the donor network, a very kind woman named Sarah. I told her about every conversation I had, and exactly what I had learned. I asked if Gery would be able to donate his corneas, optic nerves and tissues. Though she, too, was extremely sympathetic, I was disappointed again. Federal regulations prohibit Alzheimer's patients from donating any body part because they may not have Alzheimer's. They may have CJD.

Three years earlier, our lives had been altered forever by the words, "You have Alzheimer's." It was surprising to learn that the Food and Drug Administration mistrusted Gery's diagnosis.

Federal regulations prohibit Alzheimer's patients from donating body parts because Alzheimer's may be the wrong diagnosis.

I had heard of CJD on an episode of the television medical drama *House,* the source of all my really interesting medical information. Creutzfeldt-Jakob Disease is a neurological disorder, the human form of mad cow disease. It can be transmitted through blood transfusions or transplants. Some CJD symptoms resemble those of Alzheimer's. However, while early onset Alzheimer's is rare, CJD is much rarer, occurring in one in a million people.

When a doctor in his fifties has memory problems, an alarming number of people get involved in figuring out why. Gery saw multiple doctors, had every possible test including a PET scan and was finally diagnosed with Alzheimer's. Neurologists at the Mayo Clinic confirmed the diagnosis. None of Gery's doctors even hinted it might be something other than Alzheimer's.

In a few days, I called Sarah again. I described the very thorough process that led to Gery's diagnosis. I told her about Gery's brother and how strongly Gery felt about organ donation. I told her how important it was to find meaning in Gery's illness and death. To keep Gery from donating his corneas and tissues because of a one-in-a-million chance of a misdiagnosis made no sense.

I asked Sarah for the phone number of someone at the FDA. She told me she knew someone there and offered to follow up. About a week later, she called and asked me to meet her at the donor network office. When I arrived, she had wonderful news. She had arranged everything.

When Gery died, he would be immediately transported to the University of Iowa for a brain autopsy. A forensic pathologist I had worked with through the Iowa Association of County Medical Examiners agreed to do the autopsy. If the Alzheimer's diagnosis was confirmed, they would take Gery's corneas and tissues and his body would be transported back home for cremation.

There was one potential roadblock. If Gery died of septic poisoning as the result of an infection, he would be unable to donate.

At the end of our meeting, Sarah thanked me for being unwilling to accept no as a final answer to my questions.

"I learned so much in this process," she told me. "If you hadn't pressed me, that wouldn't have happened. I think your husband would be proud of you."

That was a very good day.▼

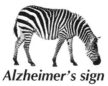

Alzheimer's sign

One night, Gery tried to get back into his clinic after hours. He put the wrong code into the digital security device so many times that an alarm was tripped at the local police station and an officer came. He wanted back in because he had left his car keys on his desk.

*Suffering among the
dying in America
is pervasive, and
so much of it is
unnecessary.*

IRA BYOCK, MD
Academy of Hospice and
Palliative Medicine

challenges a power of attorney for health care or business, the judge appoints a dispassionate third party as the new decision-maker, not the family member who mounted the challenge.

Our attorney solicited letters from doctors who had been treating Gery—a neurologist, a family physician and a psychiatrist. All three stated Gery was competent and capable of making decisions.

A videographer was hired to record a question and answer session with Gery and his subsequent signing of the legal documents. It was clearly stated in the video that I had not accompanied Gery to the office that day. Our lawyer said this was the most bulletproof power of attorney and living will he had ever done.

I met with our family physician to discuss every scenario that could arise when he reached the end stage of the illness.

I knew that, at the end of Gery's life, some family members would insist that he receive treatments he had said he didn't want, the same treatments prohibited by his living will. I decided I wouldn't share our legal documents with anyone whose motives I mistrusted. I was widely criticized for refusing to provide copies of Gery's living will, but I saw no reason to make things more difficult for myself by assisting people on a legal fishing expedition.

As I anticipated, I was repeatedly threatened with legal action. I considered Gery's last wishes to be a sacred trust and was prepared to fight back in court, but nothing came of the threats. Later, a well-respected physician who had worked with Gery's father said, "If I'm ever in a situation like Gery's, I hope someone like you is in charge."

When Gery went into long-term care, I met with our family doctor to discuss every scenario that could arise when he reached the final stage of the illness. I was determined that he would be comfortable and pain-free until the end. I was assured that pain could be managed under any circumstances.

Gery's 'don't feed me' directive caused the greatest amount of difficulty and controversy. I discussed his statement at length with the nursing home staff. As a starting point, we all agreed that no one would force feed him, a common nursing home practice in the past. After that, things got tougher. I thought long and hard about Gery's statement and talked to doctors who were also Gery's friends. His words could not have been clearer and I kept coming back to the same conclusion. Gery wanted to feed himself or not eat. This was reinforced one day when I was feeding him bites of yogurt. Gritting his teeth, he grabbed my wrist and pushed my hand away.

Understandably, the nursing home administration wanted to avoid violating the law, so we developed a compromise plan. We made sandwiches, cut them into small pieces and handed them to him. We poured liquids into a small cup and put the cup in his hand. Someone sat with him at mealtimes and reminded him to eat.

When the time came that Gery couldn't put a fork to his mouth, they fed him. By then, his dementia was so severe he couldn't have pushed anyone's hand away, but every time I saw someone feeding him, I could hear his words to me the day he was diagnosed.

People told me there were rumors around town that I was trying to starve my husband to death. Considering how much I agonized over the meaning of Gery's directive, this was vicious and unfair. It was also incredibly stupid. If starving him was my goal, I could have accomplished it with far less scrutiny by keeping him at home.

In the end, I was less concerned with silly gossip than I was with the feeling I had let Gery down. He was courageous enough to face the reality of his illness, and his directive was an attempt to preserve his dignity. In my heart, I knew that the compromise feeding plan violated his wishes. I understand why people were shocked by the idea of not feeding him; I wasn't even sure I was comfortable with it. But why did other peoples' comfort overrule Gery's wishes?

I hope Gery knows how hard I tried. There were too many people with other agendas. ▼

*True love doesn't have
a happy ending because true
love never ends. Letting go
is one way of saying
'I love you'.*

SOURCE UNKNOWN

CHAPTER 33

The love will survive

I knew it was coming, but when it finally happened I wasn't prepared. Four months before Gery went to the nursing home, we were walking in the park, he looked directly at me and asked, "Where's my wife? Where is Chris?"

I began crying but averted my face so he couldn't see. "She's running errands," I choked. "She'll be back soon."

The experts said this was the correct answer. They didn't mention that hearing this question from the man you love would feel like a knife in your heart. I couldn't help asking, "Gery, who am I?"

"I don't know," he responded, looking upset. "I just know how much I love you."

Gery and I met in the fall of our sophomore year in high school when, in the library, he tossed a note in my lap that read, "What are you doing tonight?" We dated off and on for three years but parted ways after graduation. We met again at our thirtieth class reunion at the local country club. He asked me to dance. Smiling down at me, he recalled our first kiss on the porch of my childhood home.

We were walking in the park, he looked directly at me and asked, 'Where's my wife? Where is Chris?'

"My feet didn't touch the ground on my way home," he told me. That first kiss and his last football game, he said, were his favorite memories of high school.

Nine months later, he asked me to marry him. We got married two years after that in a lovely old park in our hometown.

There were serious problems. Any second marriage faces a host of

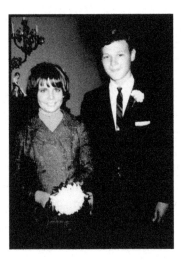

**GERY AND ME, HIGH SCHOOL
HOMECOMING DANCE, 1967**

difficult issues. I believe had it been just Gery and me, we could have worked through any problem, but Gery had additional baggage, much of which I knew nothing about until I had quit my job and moved to another state to be with him. These problems were beyond our influence and eventually, I had to face the fact we would never have a normal life in such a dysfunctional environment. I still loved him, but I gave up.

Heartbroken, I told Gery I was leaving. He put his hands on my shoulders. "I'll follow you," he said quietly. His willingness to be totally vulnerable amazed me, just as it had when we were young.

We sought counseling and we made it. Every day, Gery told me how happy he was that we were together. He was counting on us being married for at least thirty-five years.

He related a wonderful story of a couple in their late eighties who had been his patients when he was a young physician. When the gentleman died, his wife cried and said, "He was such a good lover." Gery smiled at me and said, "I hope that's us someday."

We had been married a little over five years when we learned he had early onset Alzheimer's. As the dementia marched through his brain, it was increasingly difficult for me to remember the man I fell in love with. The smart, sweet, sexy guy I married was fading from the picture, taking with him our identity as a couple.

Having a husband with Alzheimer's wreaked havoc with my emotions and my libido. In the months following his diagnosis, I was severely depressed. By the time I shook off the depression, more and more of my time was spent helping Gery with activities of daily living. I wasn't sleeping well and exhaustion took its toll. When I looked at him, I felt overwhelming pity. All libido busters.

Alzheimer's upended the dynamics of our relationship. As the disease advanced, it wasn't possible for us to relate to each other in the manner of a normal couple. We were no longer on an equal plane; there was no sharing of events, experiences or emotions. Increasingly, I was the parent and he the child. As that dynamic settled in permanently, I lost my desire for him.

We made love occasionally, but my heart wasn't in it and I felt overwhelming sadness afterward. I wish I had felt differently. On the rare occasion when the old Gery fought his way through the fog, he seemed to desire me as he always had.

On Valentine's Day in 2010, a friend helped him get me a card. Gery tried to write the same message of love he had written in many other cards. I had watched him struggle mightily just to sign his name, and the card touched me beyond words. Gery's capacity for love amazed me, just as it had when we were young.

With normalcy slipping from my grasp, I was reluctant to abandon the last vestiges of a normal marriage—sleeping together.

When he began having seizure-like episodes at night, I was advised to sleep in another bedroom so I wouldn't be injured. I spent one night in our spare bedroom. It made me so sad that I returned to our bed the next night and stayed there. With normalcy slipping from my grasp, I was reluctant to abandon the last vestiges of a normal marriage—sleeping together.

I'll always, always
have a crush on you.

Happy Birthday
You are the
Best girl
even
Love Gery

I love you
you are
Best d
Girl

BIRTHDAY CARD FROM GERY   VALENTINE FROM GERY
AUGUST, 2005   FEBRUARY, 2010

As the disease progressed, Gery's sleep patterns were increasingly erratic. He had problems falling asleep and staying asleep. Many nights, he couldn't even relax his head back onto the pillow, but lay stiffly on his back with his head raised off the bed. I tried warm milk and soothing conversation. Gery's neurologist prescribed several medications. Nothing worked.

One night when we went to bed, I maneuvered his arm around me, put my head on his shoulder and rubbed his stomach. I felt him relax. I fell asleep with my head on his shoulder, and it was almost like when we were first married. I did this often in the weeks to come. He rarely slept all night, but he slept for a few hours.

As Gery's other senses became less reliable, I touched him more. When his anxiety became unmanageable, particularly late in the afternoon, a back or neck rub seemed to help. I hugged him often and he appeared to enjoy it though I was never sure he knew who I was.

When he went to the nursing home, I encouraged the staff to touch and hug him. Experts say that even in the last stage of the disease, Alzheimer's patients respond to a gentle touch or a kind voice. Even at the end, they know if they are being treated with love and respect.

Gery's weight loss accelerated during the last year of his life, and eventually he lost so much weight that his watch was loose on his

Dr. Sutton
Wedding
Ring
_11-3-10_

wrist. One day, I noticed he wasn't wearing his wedding band. Afraid the ring would fall off and be lost, someone on the staff put it in a small envelope marked "Dr. Sutton wedding ring". I took the envelope home and angrily shoved it out of sight in a drawer. The Alzheimer's was like an unstoppable pestilence. Was there no aspect of our relationship it would leave untouched?

Seeing him in such a pitiful state for so many months began to wear on me. I wondered how much more he could deteriorate and how much longer he would suffer. I wondered if I would ever be able to remember my husband as he was before the Alzheimer's or how much I loved him.

As he had so many other times, Gery corrected my emotional course. I was visiting him one afternoon when he was having a bad day. He was mostly unresponsive. During the year he was in the nursing home, I had learned it was better to leave if I started getting upset because my tears upset him.

I wondered if I would ever be able to remember my husband as he was before the Alzheimer's, or how much I loved him.

I told him I was leaving and he surprised me by grabbing my hand and pulling me down so my face was close to his. "I just love you so much," he said, carefully enunciating every syllable. I was shocked at the clarity of his words.

"I love you, too," I choked. "Promise me you won't forget." I said this every time, but Gery rarely responded.

"I promise," he whispered, and kissed me on the cheek.

For a glorious split second, I saw the Gery I had known before the

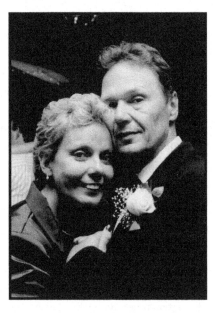

GERY AND ME
JUNE, 2008

nightmare. It was April of 2000, Boston's Logan Airport. He had invited me to watch him run the Boston Marathon. Gery had arrived in Boston earlier that day and came back to the airport to meet me. I saw him as he was in that blissful moment, jogging toward me tall and handsome, his arms reaching out. He had a huge smile on his face. I could hear him calling, "Hi, sweetheart!"

It was one of the happiest moments of my life because I loved him and we were together. I knew that no matter how long I stayed on this earth, no one would ever be that glad to see me again.

It was a miracle that this beautiful memory came back to me at that precise moment, and I vowed to keep a firm grip on it. For several years, I feared that my love for Gery had been obliterated by the horror of Alzheimer's. I couldn't have been more wrong. My love for Gery was never gone, it was always there hibernating. I knew that time would put my terrible memories of Gery's illness into the proper perspective, and the love would be resurrected when I was finally done with sadness and tears.

On that day, I knew the Alzheimer's wasn't going to beat us. ▼

No more cold iron
shackles on my feet.
I'll fly away.

ALBERT BRUMLEY
1929 gospel song
I'll Fly Away

CHAPTER 34

Our Christmas angel

On Tuesday, December 20, 2011, I spent the afternoon with Gery at the nursing home. We sat in the hospitality room, where a small group of volunteer musicians played Christmas music. It was one of Gery's good days. He appeared comfortable and relaxed.

When the concert ended, I took him to his room. I told him I was leaving town for Christmas and would see him when I returned. He didn't respond.

Though the nurses often assured me that Gery knew who I was, he hadn't called me by name for months. My daughter Kelly bears a strong resemblance to me many years ago. She had visited Gery on Thanksgiving Day a month earlier. Miraculously, when he saw her he said, "Christine." Long-term memory sometimes triumphs over advanced Alzheimer's and I was very grateful for this gift.

On that Tuesday, one last time I asked, "Do you know who I am?" His words were garbled but unmistakable. "You're the greatest." He had said this many times during our marriage.

I wondered what Gery would say, and that made me smile. I could hear him ask, as he always had, 'Can I come with you?'

I kissed him, told him I loved him and said goodbye. The next day, I drove to my daughter's house for the Christmas holiday. At eleven p.m., the nursing home staff called to tell me Gery had a low grade fever. Our family physician was monitoring his condition.

Early the next morning, I called the nursing home. Gery's nurse told me his fever was higher and he was unresponsive. I called our physician, who had been checking on Gery regularly. He said Gery had a septic infection and was "deeply unresponsive." His kidneys would shut down, probably within the next twenty-four hours. Gery was dying.

I spent the morning calling all his family members and our closest friends. Gery's sister called and told me she planned to sit with him until the others arrived.

From five hundred miles away, I wondered what I should do. I remembered my Dad saying "If you haven't settled accounts with someone by the time they're dying, it's too late."

When I was thirty-one, my Dad was admitted to the hospital on a Tuesday night and died of an aortal aneurysm in his room before I even knew he was sick. My Dad and I were kindred spirits, and I was heartbroken. Then a friend asked me, "Did you have a good relationship with your dad? Did you ever say anything to him you wish you could take back?" I answered yes to the first question, no to the second. My friend said I was very, very fortunate.

I decided to stay where I was. Gery was in a coma. There was nothing else for me to say or to prove. The others could have the deathbed scene. It was my Christmas gift to them.

I wondered what Gery would say, and that made me smile because I could hear him ask, as he always had, "Can I come with you?"

Gery died at seven a.m. on Saturday, December 24, 2011. He was sixty years and six months old. I was told he died peacefully.▼

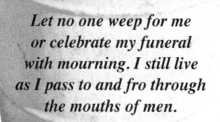

*Let no one weep for me
or celebrate my funeral
with mourning. I still live
as I pass to and fro through
the mouths of men.*

QUINTUS ENNIUS
ancient Roman poet

CHAPTER 35

Mourn a death, or celebrate a life?

In December of 2000, one of Gery's best friends—a high school classmate—died of Lou Gehrig's disease at age fifty. He left behind a wife and two teenage sons. Though his wife did her best to make the funeral service positive, it was very sad. Chuck's other friends were obviously grief-stricken, but Gery seemed OK.

He told me that his mourning process had started three years earlier when Chuck called with the news of his diagnosis.

"I came home and we all got together," Gery related. "We had a great night drinking beer and talking about the old days. I knew it was probably the last time we'd be together, but I suspected the other guys didn't understand what the diagnosis meant."

On Thursday, October 11, 2007—the worst day of my life—we learned Gery had early onset Alzheimer's. There is a river of tears between that day and the day he died four years, two months and thirteen days later.

There is a river of tears between that day and the day he died four years, two months and thirteen days later.

As Gery's partner and caregiver, I was beside him for every step of the journey. There were days when I would have traded places with just about anyone, but I didn't have the luxury of escaping or denying the reality of his illness. I mourned every day as I watched him slip further and further away.

In the fall of 2011, I sensed Gery was nearing the end, and I began thinking about how to memorialize him. Early in our marriage, we bought a plot in the local cemetery, in a row with Gery's brothers,

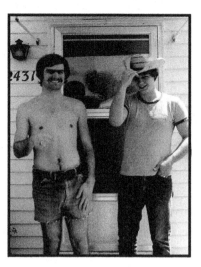

GERY (RIGHT) WITH CHUCK
Early 1970s

parents and grandparents, and a stone's throw from my parents' graves. The day we bought the plot, we decided to be cremated and buried together. Gery said he wanted his ashes to be buried so that people would have a place to visit.

During the last year of Gery's life, several of his family members told me they were dreading a difficult church funeral. I agreed. I have nothing against traditional funerals, but considering the circumstances of Gery's illness, it just didn't feel right.

It was my right and privilege to memorialize an exceptional man. When I thought about how Gery had lived, a sad church funeral seemed even less appropriate. Though he experienced more than his share of tragedy, including a fatal and incurable disease, he was also an incurable optimist. Throughout his illness, he continued to smile.

Gery was the only truly selfless person I've ever known. Because he always put everyone else's wishes ahead of his own, I wanted a memorial that put Gery in the spotlight. His choice to be cremated gave me the luxury of time to plan an event that balanced mourning his death and celebrating his life.

Our minister agreed to officiate even if the memorial wasn't held at the church. I chose a Saturday in April, a week after Easter. By then, the threat of blizzards is mostly over. The time gap would make it possible for Gery's out-of-state family and friends to attend. I decided to have two separate memorials that Saturday—a traditional graveside service in the morning and, in the evening, a celebration of Gery's life. Planning Gery's memorial was cathartic and rewarding. I reconnected with him in ways I never could have anticipated.

I rented a facility that is normally used for wedding receptions and class reunions. At my daughter's suggestion, I planned a meal of Gery's favorite foods. Gery was a saver, and in his storage tubs I found many items for a memorabilia display. My friends arranged the display and, when I saw it, I was impressed anew with all Gery had accomplished in the sixty years he was granted.

Purple is the color of Alzheimer's awareness, and many of us wore purple to the celebration. I made centerpieces with pictures of Gery and table favors with the words "Memories Matter." I printed flyers with information about Alzheimer's.

Planning Gery's memorial was cathartic and rewarding. I reconnected with him in ways I never could have anticipated.

Though anyone was welcome to share memories of Gery, I asked certain people to speak because they represented particular phases of his life. I asked his sister to talk about their childhood. One of our high school classmates who played on the football team with Gery collected memories from their teammates. I asked a college friend to talk about Gery's days in undergraduate school. One of his colleagues agreed to talk about Gery's career as a physician and the number of lives he touched.

Several years ago I saw an interview with documentary filmmaker Ken Burns. He said his starting point for a new film isn't the photos, but the music. The music for Gery's memorial was the first item on my planning agenda. During the time Gery was in the nursing home,

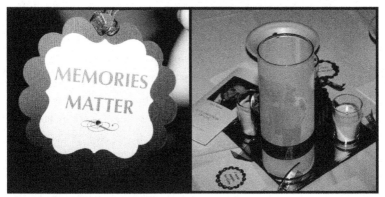

TABLE FAVOR AND CENTERPIECE   Photos by Traci Clark
Gery's Celebration of Life

I saw him react with unbridled joy twice—when I brought Lucy to
see him and when the hospice music therapist sang "Somewhere
Over the Rainbow", one of his favorite songs.

I asked a friend to sing "Abide With Me" at the graveside service
because it was sung at the funerals of my grandmother and great
grandmother. I asked three friends from choir to sing "God Be With
You Till We Meet Again" on Saturday evening because this song
was sung at the funeral of Gery's grandmother.

I wanted one upbeat song, and chose "I'll Fly Away", a great old
hymn about dying and going to heaven. A bluegrass version of the
song was on the soundtrack of the movie "Oh Brother Where Art
Thou?" Gery loved the movie and bought the soundtrack.

One of my best friends, my singing partner since we were thirteen,
took responsibility for this song. Kim and her husband found
mandolin and guitar players. Our minister's husband, an insurance
underwriter by day and bass player by night, agreed to join the band
as did another friend who is an accomplished pianist. Kim, her
husband, her daughter and I did the vocals. We rehearsed once, just
three hours before the memorial began. I knew Gery was lending a
hand. I've never heard a song come together with so little rehearsal.

I also included recorded music in the celebration. I had a list of
Gery's favorite songs and hired a professional to turn them into a

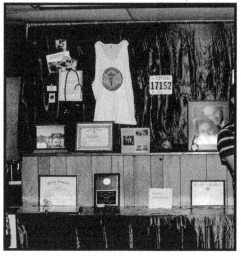

**GERY'S
MEMORABILIA
DISPLAY**

fifteen-minute medley. This became the background music for a
slide show of Gery's life I created on my Mac. Gery's sisters and
other family members provided many of the photos.

In the months before Gery died, I wondered if the image of Gery
in the final stage of Alzheimer's would be burned into my memory
forever. Sifting through those photos, arranging and rearranging the
images I chose for the slide show, I got the answer to my question.
The photos evoked laughter, tears and a myriad of other emotions.
They reacquainted me with the boy and the man I had known and
loved. The awful picture of a once vital man ravaged by Alzheimer's
began to fade.

When Gery and I began attending church, I joined the choir and
was sometimes asked to do a solo. Gery loved hearing me sing. I can
still see him sitting in the pew, smiling up at me. I wanted to sing for
Gery's memorial but I knew I wouldn't be able to sing a solo that
night. My solution was to prerecord a song, accompanied by a dear
friend who often played for me.

I choose "The Blessing" by the group Celtic Woman. It was on a
CD Gery gave me for Saint Patrick's Day in 2005. Most people
believe the song is a mother's message to her child. For me, in the

context of Gery's illness, it's about watching over someone you love.

Recording the song was difficult but I did my best. I used it as background music for a brief slide show featuring pictures of Gery and me. It was a nice addition to the celebration, but I could never have anticipated it would lead to a miracle.

A week after I recorded the song, I visited the high school to talk with someone about establishing a scholarship in Gery's name. I walked through the halls and down memory lane. This was where Gery and I met when we were young, carefree and full of promise.

I was thinking of those golden days as I approached the choral music room. Incredibly, as I reached the open doorway, I heard the opening chords of "The Blessing". I looked inside and saw a girl at the piano. She began singing, her voice breathy and beautiful. I was stunned. If my song had been "Amazing Grace", I wouldn't have thought twice about the coincidence. But this song?

I knew Gery was there. He was letting me know he's OK.

There was a downpour the night of Gery's celebration, but well over two hundred people came. People smiled and laughed through their tears. Everyone sang along when we played "I'll Fly Away". They sang for Gery, and it was a wonderful moment.

Many people told me it was exactly the kind of memorial they want for themselves. I hope the celebration will help people remember Gery and his wonderful life, and remind them that they were better for knowing him. I especially appreciated a friend who said, "The amount of love in that room was amazing."

Did you hear that, sweetie? I hope so.▼

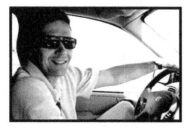

A final word

Gery's death was a blessing in light of his suffering, but that does little to ease my acute sense of loss.

Two weeks after he died, I went to the basement to begin the sad task of sorting through his memorabilia. The first item I pulled at random from a box was a greeting card I sent to Gery in 1967 when I was on vacation in California. I had forgotten about the card and, of course, had no idea he'd saved it all these years. I started to cry, returned the card to the box and went back upstairs.

In the months following Gery's death, I began final editing of this book. As I worked, forgotten details of his illness began filtering back. For example, I recalled a dreadful day shortly after we learned Gery had Alzheimer's, the day we went to collect personal items from his office at the clinic. For over four years, these hours of utter despair were completely blocked from my memory.

The human mind is a wondrous thing. Our memories of the most painful events are not allowed entrance until we have regained our ability to process them. More proof that time is the best healer.

Our memories of the most painful events are not allowed entrance until we have regained our ability to process them.

I'm encouraged by the fact that, with each passing week, I cry less often. I am busy with my freelance business and other projects. I continue the search for meaning in Gery's illness and death.

I would be happy to receive feedback or questions from readers. Please email me at **caregiver822@gmail.com.**

A paperback copy of this book can be purchased through the CreateSpace eStore (www.createspace.com/3885391) or on Amazon.com, which also has the Kindle version. ▼

Acknowledgments

This quote from Russell Lynes, former editor of Harper's Magazine, is one of my favorites: *Every journalist has a novel inside him, which is an excellent place for it.*

I was never one of those journalists who believed I had a novel inside me. Throughout my career, my focus has been writing about other people. I've always worked for a salary and on a schedule. I've learned that writing about my own life—with no paycheck or deadline ahead—is the literary equivalent of working without a net.

I am fortunate to have a network of people who were ready to catch me when I fell. Without them, I may never have finished this book. I'll be forever grateful to:

My daughter Kelly, who loved her stepfather without an agenda, cherishes his ugly, out-of-date winter coat and understood when I couldn't always be there for her. My son-in-law Skyler, who proposed to Kelly in our living room a month after Gery's diagnosis and made me smile when I thought I would never smile again.

My son Nathan, who worries about me too much and will always be my favorite sounding board and sous chef. My daughter-in-law Traci, who shot many of the photos for this book and, when my caregiving burden was heaviest, said "Call me anytime you need to talk, even if it's the middle of the night."

The Steel Magnolias—Gery called us "YaYa Girls"—Connie, Davi, DeDe, Holly, Kim and Susan. My sisters-in-spirit who cried with me, supported me, defended me and kept me from going crazy. Holly shared my early draft with her book club, encouraged me to dig deeper and greatly improved my book with her Photoshop and proofreading skills.

My dear friend and business partner Cheri Jensen, who was wise enough to marry her high school sweetheart the first time around, and had the perfect business idea at the perfect time.

My grandchildren Hayden, Noah and Scarlett, a source of true joy and hope for the future. ▼

Resources

The Internet contains a prodigious amount of information on every aspect of Alzheimer's disease and caregiving. If the web site address ends in .**org** it's usually a site sponsored by a non-profit organization. If it ends in .**com** it's sponsored by a commercial entity. That doesn't necessarily mean the information is suspect. (For example, the Mayo Clinic's website ends in .com, but the information is written by top professionals in the field.) If the web address ends in .**gov**, it's a site sponsored by a local, state or government agency.

All the resources I list here are electronic sources because it is the most convenient medium for caregivers. Even if you are looking for a book or a DVD, your starting point should be a computer. Book sites such as Amazon.com provide lists of books by topic, and valuable reader reviews of each book.

If you don't have access to a computer or aren't computer literate, ask someone to research Alzheimer's topics and download articles. In my experience, people want to help, and this would be a great way to do it.

Some Alzheimer's web sites contain message boards and blogs for patients and caregivers. These forums provide a valuable opportunity to communicate with others in your situation.

Alzheimer's websites

The Alzheimer's Association—**alz.org**. On the home page, click on "I am a caregiver". Valuable information, message boards and a 24/7 helpline, 800.272.3900. Free Alzheimer's E-newsletter.

The Alzheimer's Reading Room—**alzheimersreadingroom.com.** This blog was created by Bob DeMarco, caregiver for his mother. Over 3,400 articles on every aspect of Alzheimer's and Alzheimer's caregiving.

The National Alliance for Caregiving—**caregiving.org**. Support and information for family caregivers.

The Alzheimer's Foundation of America—**alzfdn.org**. Information and services for anyone confronting dementia. Latest scientific developments. Free e-newsletter.

The Mayo Clinic—**mayoclinic.com/health/alzheimers-disease/ DS00161**. Articles on Alzheimer's topics written by Mayo Clinic staff. Free Alzheimer's e-newsletter, blog for caregivers.

US Department of Health and Human Services—**alzheimers.gov**. Support and information for family caregivers. First phase of a federal government plan to find an effective treatment for Alzheimer's by 2025. Links to government agencies and organizations.

WebMD—**webmd.com/alzheimers/default.htm**. Comprehensive information on a wide variety of Alzheimer's-related topics. Reader reviews of Alzheimer's medications.

Alzheimer's Disease Education and Referral Center—**alzheimers.org**. Information on Alzheimer's disease research, diagnosis, treatment, drugs, clinical trials, and federal programs and resources.

Alzheimer's Research Forum—**alzforum.org**. Compendium of information for researchers, physicians and the public. News, discussion forums, directory of drugs and clinical trials, and research advances.

Signs of Alzheimer's

The difference between normal memory loss and memory loss resulting from Alzheimer's disease. Alzheimer's Association, 2009. **alz.org/ alzheimers_disease_10_signs_of_alzheimers.asp#typical**

A list of 34 Alzheimer's symptoms and explanations of the different types of Alzheimer's. Other diseases that cause the same symptoms. Rightdiagnosis.com, HealthGrades Inc., 2011. **rightdiagnosis.com/a/ alzheimers_disease/symptoms.htm#symptom_list**

How Alzheimer's affects the brain

Interactive tour of the brain, including a lay person's explanation of how the brain works and how Alzheimer's affects it. The Alzheimer's Association, 2012. **alz.org/alzheimers_disease_4719.asp**

"The Alzheimer's Brain" by Christine Kennard. About.com, 2005. **alzheimers.about.com/od/caregivers/a/alz_brain.htm**

Alzheimer's risk factors

"Determining Your Risk Factors for Alzheimer's Disease" by Dennis Thompson, Jr., EverydayHealth.com, 2009. **everydayhealth.com/ alzheimers/alzheimers-risk-factors.aspx**

"Alzheimer's genes: Are you at risk?" by Mayo Clinic staff, 2010. **mayoclinic.com/health/alzheimers-genes/AZ00047**

"Genetic Risk Factors". No author listed. Fisher Center for Alzheimer's Research Foundation. **alzinfo.org/07/about_alzheimers/genetic-risk-factors**

Stages of Alzheimer's

"Seven Stages of Alzheimer's". No author listed. The Alzheimer's Association, 2012. **alz.org/alzheimers_disease_stages_of_alzheimers.asp**

"Stages of Alzheimer's" by Barry Reisberg, MD, Fisher Center for Alzheimer's Research Foundation, 2012. **alzinfo.org/clinical-stages-of-alzheimers**

Alzheimer's medications

"Evaluating Prescription Drugs Used to Treat Alzheimer's Disease: Comparing Effectiveness, Safety, and Price". No author listed. Consumer Reports, updated in 2012. **consumerreports.org/health/resources/pdf/ best-buy-drugs/AlzheimersFINAL.pdf**

"Current Alzheimer's Treatments". No author listed. The Alzheimer's Association, 2012. **alz.org/research/science/alzheimers_disease_ treatments.asp.**

Clinical trials

"Understanding Clinical Trials". No author listed. US National Institutes of Health, 2007. **clinicaltrials.gov/ct2/info/understand**

Clinical Trials for Alzheimer's Disease—Alzheimer's Association Trial Match. **alz.org/research/clinical_trials/find_clinical_trials_ trialmatch.asp**

Long Term Care

"Alzheimer's: Consider options for long term care" by Mayo Clinic staff. Mayoclinic.com, 2010. **mayoclinic.com/health/alzheimers/AZ00028**

"Dementia and Alzheimer's care—Planning and preparing for the road ahead" by Doug Russell, Tina de Benedictus and Joanna Saisan, 2012. Helpguide.org. **helpguide.org/elder/alzheimers_disease_dementias_ caring_caregivers.htm#considering**

Managing Alzheimer's behaviors

"Managing Unpredictable Behavior in People with Alzheimer's Disease". No author listed. WebMD, 2012. **webmd.com/alzheimers/guide/ managing-unpredictable-behavior**

"Behavior Management: How to Manage the Challenging Behaviors of Alzheimer's Disease" by Carrie Hill, PhD. About.com, 2008. **alzheimers.about.com/od/caregiving/a/behaviors.htm**

Alzheimer's and driving

"When should patients with Alzheimer's stop driving?" by Deniz Erten-Lyons, MD. Neurology, 2008. **neurology/org/content/70/14/e45.long**

"At the Crossroads: Family Conversations about Alzheimer's Disease, Dementia and Driving." No author listed. The Hartford, 2010. **hartfordauto.thehartford.com/UI/Downloads/Crossroads.pdf**

Alzheimer's financial and legal issues

"Prepare for the Financial Impact of Alzheimer's" by Susan Garland, editor, Kiplinger's Retirement Report, 2012. **kiplinger.com**

"Alzheimer's Disease Financial Planning". No author listed. MedicineNet.com. **medicinenet.com/financial_planning_in_alzheimers_ disease/article.htm**

"Alzheimer's Disease and Legal Issues". No author listed. WebMD, 2012. **webmd.com/alzheimers/guide/legal-issues**

"The Alzheimer's Legal Survival Kit" by elder law attorney Michael J. Young. (Some information is specific to California.) **walnutcreekelderlaw. com/TheAlzheimersLegalSurvivalKit.html**

End-of-life issues

"Late Stage and End-of-life Care: Caregiving in the final stages of life" by Melissa Wayne, MA, Lawrence Robinson and Jeanne Segal, PhD. HelpGuide.org, updated 2012. **helpguide.org/elder alzheimers_disease_ dementia_caring_final_stage.htm**

"Late Stage Care". No author listed. The Alzheimer's Association, 2012. **alz.org/nyc/in_my_community_17737.asp**

"Alzheimer's disease: Anticipating end-of-life needs" by Mayo Clinic staff. The Mayo Clinic, 2011. **mayoclinic.com/health/alzheimers/ HQ00618**

Stress, Burnout, Depression and Guilt:
A Caregiver's Emotional Well-being

"Why Being a Caregiver is So Hard" by Sharon O'Brien for About.com. **seniorliving.about.com/od/healthnutrition/a/caregiverstips.htm**

"Recognizing Caregiver Burnout". No author listed. WebMD.com. **webmd.com/caregiver-recognizing-burnout**

"Tips for coping with Caregiver Stress", reviewed by Louise Chang, MD. WebMD.com, 2012. **webmd.com/balance/stress-management/ caregiver-advice-cope**

"7 Depression Busters for Caregivers" by Therese Borchard, Associate Editor, PsychCentral.com, 2010. **psychcentral.com/blog/archives/ 2010/02/24/7-depression-busters-for-caregivers/**

"Caregiver Depression: Prevention Counts", Mayo Clinic staff, 2010. **mayoclinic.com/health/caregiver-depression/MY01264**

"Caregiver Guilt—Memory and Alzheimer's Disease." Peter Rabins, MD of Johns Hopkins interviews caregivers, 2011. Transcript and video. **hopkinsmedicine.org/rabins_alzheimers**

"Feel at Peace: Lose the Caregiver Guilt", "Ten Caregiver Confessions: Secrets we aren't proud of" by Carol Bradley Bursack, AgingCare.com. **agingcare.com/Articles/**

General interest topics

"Reagan helped remove stigma of Alzheimer's" by Mary Brophy Marcus, USA Today, 2011. **usatoday.com/news/washington/2011-01-23-ronald-reagan-alzheimers_N.htm**

"What's ahead in the Alzheimer's Research Pipeline?" by Dennis Thompson Jr, reviewed by Pat Bass III, MD, MS, MPH. Everyday Health. **everydayhealth.com/alzheimers/alzheimers-research-and-future-treatments.aspx**

"Early Onset Alzheimer's Disease". No author listed. Wikipedia, the Free Encyclopedia. **en.wikipedia.org/wiki/Early-onset_Alzheimer's_disease**

"Alzheimer's Facts and Figures". No author listed. Alzheimer's Association, 2012. **alz.org/alzheimers_disease_facts_and_figures.asp**

"Alzheimer's Conference Calendar". Compiled by the Alzheimer's Research Forum. **alzforum.org/res/res/conf/default.asp**

About the author

Christine McMahon Sutton grew up in Iowa and is a graduate of the University of Iowa in Iowa City. She was a news reporter until 1986, when she joined the staff of the Iowa Medical Society in West Des Moines. At IMS, she was vice president of communications and editor of Iowa Medicine.

She was an editor and health care writer for Oklahoma Magazine in Tulsa from 2001-2006.

In 2006, she wrote the historical text One Hundred Years of Medicine in Oklahoma, which was published in the Oklahoma State Medical Association Journal on the occasion of that state's centennial. She also wrote historical articles for the Oklahoma Dental Association Journal.

In 2009, Christine and her former co-worker Cheri Jensen founded Management and Event Services, a home-based company that provides administrative services for the Iowa Association of County Medical Examiners, the Iowa Association of Pathologists and the Iowa Society of Allergy, Asthma and Immunology.

Christine has two children and three grandchildren. She and her dog Lucy live quietly in a small town in Iowa.▼